**This Book
Belongs To:**

Ms. Carletta Mitchell
26 West Line Avenue
Vauxhall, NJ 07088

WHAT DID THE DOCTOR JUST SAY?

How to Understand What Your Doctor Is
Saying and Prevent Medical Errors From
Happening to You and Your Loved Ones

Dear Carlette: Let Me Inspire You
Just A Little Higher

1.16.2013

Lynn R. Parker,
Registered Nurse, Nurse Practitioner, Patient Advocate

iUniverse, Inc.
New York   Bloomington

What Did The Doctor Just Say?
How to Understand What Your Doctor Is Saying and Prevent
Medical Errors From Happening to You and Your Loved Ones

Copyright © 2009 Lynn R. Parker

The information in this book is not intended to act as or be a substitute for
medical advice or treatment. It is intended only, to enhance communication
and understanding between doctors, patients, and other healthcare
providers, thereby increasing patient safety. Neither the author nor the
publisher of this book endorses the use of the information in this book
as a treatment guide or as a substitute for seeking medical advice.

iUniverse books may be ordered through booksellers or by contacting:

iUniverse
1663 Liberty Drive
Bloomington, IN 47403
www.iuniverse.com
1-800-Authors (1-800-288-4677)

Because of the dynamic nature of the Internet, any Web addresses or
links contained in this book may have changed since publication and
may no longer be valid. The views expressed in this work are solely those
of the author and do not necessarily reflect the views of the publisher,
and the publisher hereby disclaims any responsibility for them.

ISBN: 978-0-595-52909-4 (pbk)
ISBN: 978-0-595-62959-6 (ebk)

Printed in the United States of America

iUniverse rev. date: 11/23/09

To My Creator

You have always been and will always be the guiding light that lives deep inside of me and I Love You.

TABLE OF CONTENTS

Acknowledgements

This book would not have been possible without the contributions of my Mother, Olivia Parker Daniels. As I look back over the last years of my Mothers life I realize that I was given two very precious gifts during that time. I was given the honor of caring for my Mom when she needed me, and I was granted the time and space needed to write this book. That time and this book are a very important part of my Mothers legacy to me and to everyone who is helped by this work. I directly tribute any success this book enjoys to the time I spent with my Mother during the last days of her life, time for which I am deeply grateful.

To my children Khalil and Olivia, your unwavering faith in me gave me the confidence I needed to persevere.

To my sister, Harriett, your words never fail to hearten me or to let me know I'm on the right track. Thank you for your insights into me and my work. Insights only you could have, because only you have been there my entire lifetime and for that I love you and I thank you.

To my cousin April, who believes in me like no one else and always comes when I call for help, for that I thank you and I love you Cousin Sister Girl.

To my Dear, Dear, Friend Sharon who has helped me through the most challenging times of my life, without your support I truly don't know if I would have made it. Thank you so very much for always being there.

To Maxine, though whose eyes I acquired a vision of myself that has empowered me with the self-esteem necessary to accomplish all of my hopes and dreams. For that vision I can never repay you and I will always love and respect you.

And to my students, my patients and everyone else who gave me your love and encouragement over the last two years. Without your kind words and prayers I'm not sure I would have been able to complete this project. I love each of you for the special gifts only you could have given me. Thank you and May God bless and keep you all in His loving care.

Lynn aka Miss Parker

INTRODUCTION

Medical errors—the mistakes made by doctors, patients, and other healthcare providers —are the fifth leading cause of death in America. Medical errors take the lives of more than 100,000 patients annually; the equivilant of thirty 9/11 bombings. Medical errors go onto injure, disable, and bankrupt another two million patients. Those injuries cost our nation's healthcare system an estimated $37.6 billion dollars per year.

The patients who experience the fewest number of medical errors and are most satisfied with the treatments they receive are those who actively participate in making their healthcare decisions. However, being an active participant in the decision making process is very difficult for a great many patients. Ninety million Americans, regardless of their level of education, have difficulty understanding what their doctor says. When patients do not understand what their doctors are saying, it is nearly impossible to take an active role in their care, and when patients are not actively involved in the process, errors are more likely occur.

According to a 2003 study conducted by the Office of the

Surgeon General, patients with little or no understanding of medical language—otherwise known as "low healthcare literacy"—tend to be sicker, they experience more medical errors, and they receive an overall inferior level care when compared to patients who have greater healthcare literacy. It is estimated that low healthcare literacy leads to nearly $73 billion dollars in extra healthcare costs every year.

What Did the Doctor Just Say? was written to help everyone increase their level of healthcare literacy and thereby be safer when entering the healthcare system. It accomplishes this by teaching patients to how to speak and understand the language of medical professionals and by teaching patients how to participate in making medical decisions.

The organizations leading the way in healthcare safety reform, organizations like the Joint Commission, The Agency for Healthcare Research and Quality, and The Institute of Medicine agree that one of the best ways to learn how to make medical decisions and to ensure patient safety, is to teach patients how to question their providers. Questions encourage interactive conversations and the exchange of helpful information. Questions help patients and providers develop partnerships based on mutual goals. Questions encourage providers to think deeply about their actions before simply performing them in routine ways. When patients ask questions, providers know they must be on their best behavior because the patient knows a thing or two and is monitoring their actions. Most importantly, questions can help the patient and the provider develop an open line of communication, and when there is open communication, patients receive better and safer care.

The questions in this book were formulated by reviewing the questions The Joint Commission, The Institute of Medicine, and The Agency for Healthcare Research and Quality recommend patients ask their providers to evaluate their treatment options. I combined those questions with questions patients have asked me over the last 20 years of my practice that did not appear on those sites. After gathering the questions I added explanations to them to help you understand why you need the answers to those questions. When you gain insight into why you need an answer you will then be able to create your own questions, questions that fit your unique situation. Once you have the answers to the questions in this book you will be able to:

- Understand your disease process.

- Learn about the most up-to-date and safest treatment plans.

- Become fully informed and make safer decisions for you and your loved ones.

This book will teach you to do all of these things and more. In doing so, it could help to save your life.

HOW TO USE THIS BOOK

Many sections in this book include questions designed to guide you through talking with your doctor and gaining valuable information during each phase of the healthcare process. Before going to the doctor or any other healthcare provider's office, become familiar with the questions you need for that visit. If, for example, you need information about your diagnosis and treatment options, view the question set titled "Understanding Your Diagnosis and Treatment Options."

Make a copy of the questions and take them with you to the visit. You or the provider can write the answers to your questions on the question worksheets you will find in the Appendix of this book. When the answers are written down, you will be able to share them with other members of *YOUR* Healthcare Team. The answers to your questions will be of great value when going for a second opinion and when you simply want to explain what the doctor said to your family members and friends. Or if you simply want to review them at your leisure they will be there for you. The very best thing about having answers is that it will go a long way toward helping you understand what the doctor just said and getting the kind of care you want and deserve. Knowing the answers to the questions will also help you to take control of your healthcare and your safety. Make as many copies as you like of the question sheets and take them with you to all of your medical visits and let your doctors know you are making their answers a part of your medical record, as this will encourage them to give you complete and accurate information.

CHAPTER ONE:

You Could be Injured or Killed by our Healthcare System

"Fear is the father of courage and the mother of safety."

Henry H. Tweedy

The Facts and Figures

If the Centers for Disease Control counted medical errors as a cause of death, they would be the fifth leading cause of death in America, taking more lives than motor vehicle accidents, breast cancer, and AIDS combined. Medical errors and stories of personal tragedy that accompany these accounts are seemingly endless. Just listen to the nightly news and you'll hear stories of medication errors that leave patients near death; surgeries performed on the wrong patients; and hospital-acquired infections that kill more than 90,000 people each year.

Sadly, for many of you reading this, medical error is not

just something you've heard about. In fact, 42 percent of surveyed patients stated they or their family members had been injured by a medical error. Statistically, each of us has a two in five-or a 40 percent-chance of being harmed by a medical error each time we enter the healthcare system.

HealthGrades, our nation's leading reviewer of healthcare quality, found that for the years 2002-04, 1.24 million errors were made while caring for hospitalized Medicare patients in the sixteen categories of error they investigated. Those errors resulted in deaths of 304,702 senior citizens. Of those deaths, 250,246 (82 percent) were potentially preventable. All totaled, these errors cost patients and taxpayers $9.3 billion dollars.

When you read the number "304,702" keep in mind it represents only *in-hospital Medicare patients*. The numbers do not include medical errors involving anyone under age 65, nor do they include medical errors that occur in doctors' offices, pharmacies, rehabilitation, or long-term care facilities. No one knows how many medical errors or deaths from errors there really are. The authors of the HealthGrades study tell us that the numbers in their report "represent only the tip of the medical-errors iceberg."

There are several reasons why we will never know just how bad things really are. The primary reason we will never know the truth may be that it is not a part of medical culture to admit wrongdoing. A 2008 University of Iowa study found only 18 percent of physicians surveyed had ever reported a minor error and only 4 percent had reported a major error.

And then there's the god syndrome. Patients and medical professionals tend to view doctors as godlike figures. When a doctor admits to an error he risks losing his godlike status and "falling from grace." Sadly, when one possesses a godlike status, it can very damaging to admit making an error.

In addition to a potential loss of status, doctors face the possibility of having to pay large settlements and losing their licenses if found guilty of causing a medical error. With so much at stake, it is understandable why doctors do not report a medical errors.

Beyond incomplete reporting by doctors, hospitals and government agencies have failed to establish a comprehensive method of reporting medical errors and calculating their costs. According to the Agency for Healthcare Research and Quality (AHRQ), the exact number of facilities that track and record medical errors and the types of errors they report cannot be documented with any degree of accuracy.

Under our current system, The Joint Commission mandates virtually every hospital in the country report life threatening errors. In contrast error reporting for non-life threatening errors is neither uniform or consistent from one facility to another. Hospital A may collect and report error statistics on falls, while Hospital B may collect and report data on medication errors. In addition, the type of errors reported and criteria for reporting them vary from state to state. As of late 2009, only twenty six states had laws that required hospitals to report medical errors. Each of these states collects data independently and is not required to share or compare findings with other reporting states.

No matter what the actual numbers are, they do not begin to convey the real meaning embedded within them. Numbers cannot convey the depth of a patients' distress when he realizes he has lost the ability to work and will soon be bankrupt due to medical costs. How can numbers convey the sadness one feels when a marriage ends under the strain of a prolonged illness? And numbers cannot begin to express the anger, depression, and resentment felt when a person's life is ruined by a healthcare system they once trusted. The numbers are big and they are bad and yet they do not begin to tell the whole story of medical error.

Your Insurance Carrier May Not Cover the Damages

Not only could you or your loved ones fall victim to a medical error, your insurance company may not pay for the care you need because of your injuries. As of October 2008, in an attempt to force hospitals to improve care and to save money, the Centers for Medicare and Medicaid Services (CMS) will no longer reimburse hospitals for a group of errors called "never events." They are so-called because it is believed these events should not and would not happen if doctors and hospitals followed established protocols designed to prevent them. Because of these beliefs the CMS no longer pays for care required after a patient is injured by a eight types of "never events."

Eight of the 28 types of errors classified as never events are responsible for the spending of approximately $22 billion Medicare dollars each year, and those eight types of errors are the first to be excluded from payment. This group of errors includes: infections from catheters (IV and Foley catheters); pressure ulcers (bedsores); air embolisms; being given the wrong type of blood; repeat surgeries needed to remove objects left inside the patient following surgery; falls; injury or death from medications, and the post operative deaths of low risk surgical patients.

Non-payment for the care required after a never event could have devastating effects on both patients and hospitals. If, for example, you develop a pressure ulcer (a bedsore), the treatment of that ulcer may require bandages, packing, antibiotics, creams, and surgery, easily costing hundreds of dollars per day. While you are in the hospital, the hospital is required to absorb the cost of caring for your injury. Once you are discharged from the hospital you may be responsible for the costs. This will depend upon the arrangement your hospital has with Medicare or your private insurance carrier, this is because recently, Blue Cross/Blue Shield, Aetna, and Cigna have announced plans to restructure their policies to deny payment of never events as well.

When you consider that Medicare alone spends up to $22 billion dollars annually to treat these eight never events, you can well imagine that thousands of patients will not be able to afford the care they need after being injured by a never event without help from their insurance carriers.

We May All Have Less Access to Healthcare

Before the instatement of the never rules, most patients had no idea that the development of a bedsore while in the hospital could be considered negligence or that they may be entitled to compensation for their pain and suffering. As a part of the never event regulations, doctors are required to inform patients they have fallen victim to a never event. With more patients being made aware they have been injured by the medical system, the number of lawsuits could skyrocket, leading to increasing malpractice rates, which some doctors and hospitals will not be able to pay. The consequences of this could be that that we'll have less access to care as doctors leave their practices and hospitals close under the financial burden of decreased reimbursements and ever increasing malpractice premiums. In fact this is already happening in some states.

With more hospitals closing, remaining emergency rooms

will be overcrowded. There are already long waits to get into surviving hospitals, where workers are exhausted from dealing with high volumes of patients. So, while the CMS may be well intentioned, the consequences of refusing to pay for never events could be tough on all of us. Fewer doctors and massive hospital closures present a very serious problem; we don't have anywhere else to go.

Now that we are aware of some of the problems in healthcare and we know that we are all at risk of falling victim to a medical error, each of us who cares about our healthcare and our safety must ask ourselves a question, and that question is: "What can I do to protect myself and my loved ones from a medical error?" Keep reading and I'll tell you.

Chapter Two

Take Charge

"A wise man ought to realize that his health is his most valuable possession and learn how to treat his illnesses by his own judgment."

Hippocrates (460-377 BC)

Why You Need to Be in Charge

At this point, you may be asking, "How can I take charge of my healthcare? I don't understand anything about medicine, and half of the time I don't understand what the doctor is saying! Besides, it's the doctor's job to be in control of my care."

If you are thinking any or all of these thoughts, you are not alone. Difficulties understanding what the doctor says and believing that it is the doctor's responsibility to make our healthcare decisions are *huge* barriers to receiving high quality healthcare. If you believe these things you will accept whatever care the doctor prescribes whether or not it meets your with expectations or your individual needs and it doesn't have to be that way. Patients who participate in making their healthcare decisions experience fewer medical errors and are happier with the care they receive. Thus, it is of vital importantance to your health and your happiness that you take charge and become the leader of **YOUR** Healthcare Team. To do this, you will need to fully debunk the myths that have taught us that the doctor should be in control of making our healthcare decisions. Let's get started.

Myth Number One: Doctors are godlike figures, more than mere mortals.

Reality: Doctors are human beings, they are not gods. They have flaws like the rest of us. Doctors are not perfect or all-knowing and the number of medical errors that occur each and every day make this fact abundantly clear.

Myth Number Two: My doctor knows best and is responsible for making my healthcare decisions.

Reality: A typical day for a doctor might start at 5:00 a.m. when he is; off to the hospital by six to see patients. At the hospital the doctor will review medical findings; see patients; write orders in charts; and collaborate with other medical professionals. Then it's time for office hours.

With a 30 percent shortage in primary care physicians

and ever decreasing insurance reimbursements, a doctor may have hundreds of patients on his roster and need to see thirty or more patients per day to financially sustain his practice. At the office, in addition to seeing patients, doctors have to take telephone calls from insurance companies, nurses, case managers, patients, and the pharmacy. And they have their own lives to manage as well. Doctors are under tremendous pressure. It is not realistic to believe your doctor can make all of your healthcare decisions with your individual needs in mind, when he may not even remember who you are.

You, on the other hand, know all of your symptoms and how you've responded to the treatments you've tried. That self-knowledge uniquely qualifies you to help your doctor make the right diagnosis and develop the best treatment plan for you.

The only way to ensure the choices made are the best ones for you is to be actively involved in making those choices. The best way to make a medical decision is to listen to what your doctor says, then to gather information from independent sources (more on this later). After you have evaluated the information you gathered and discussed the risks and benefits of each of your choices, you and your caregivers will be prepared to make treatment decisions that meet your medical needs and are in alignment with your lifestyle choices. Besides, it's not even fair to put the pressure of making all your healthcare choices on your doctors-after all they are only human!

Myth Number 3: Only the doctor knows enough to make my healthcare choices

Reality: At this point many of you do not have enough knowledge to question or to challenge your doctor's opinions, and that's okay. Everyone is challenged by all there is to know in medicine, even your doctors. Think about this: if your heart doctor went to see his diabetes doctor, he would have to learn new information regarding his care. After all, your doctor specializes in the care of the heart and may not be up-to-date on the latest treatments for diabetes. Only after some investigation could he make fully informed decisions about the care of his diabetes. Anytime anyone enters a new area of healthcare, there will be new things to learn.

However there are tools to help you obtain the information you need to participate in the decision making process and those tools will help you to make well informed safe healthcare decisions. The rest of this book is dedicated to teaching you how to effectively use those tools and to debunking the "fourth" myth: "*I could never know enough to take charge of my healthcare.*" Let's get started.

Communication is Key

According to the Joint Commission our nation's largest healthcare accrediting body, regardless of their level of education, 40-90 million Americans find medical consent forms and simple treatment directions difficult, if not impossible, to understand. An inability and/or difficulty understanding medical language is known as a low level of healthcare literacy, and a great many Americans suffer with this condition. The high school graduate, the schoolteacher, and the mechanical engineer may all find medical information difficult to understand.

At the heart of health *literacy* is a conversation that happens between the doctor and the patient. If you do not understand what the doctor is saying, you will give permission for tests, procedures, and surgeries without fully understanding the consequences of your actions. If you don't understand how to prepare for a test and you "do something wrong," the test will yield inaccurate results. You may then have to repeat the tests, which will cost more time and money, and worse yet, you could be prescribed the wrong treatments based upon your inaccurate test results.

Clearly, it is important that the doctor and patient understand one another. However, the doctor and his patient often do not understand one another and the misunderstandings begin as soon as the two meet. Does the following scenario sound familiar to you?

Doctor: "Good morning Mrs. Jones. I have read your chart and see you have a contusion in the area of your left occipital lobe, which you sustained last night after an episode of transient ataxia without any other associated symptoms and no prior history of ataxia? You are here today because you have pain in the area of your occipital lobe, which is radiating to your right temporal lobe. You are also experiencing blurred vision and a pounding headache, is that right?"

Unless you are a trained in a health-related profession, you probably thought to yourself, "What did he just say?" You probably caught on when he said, "You're here today with a complaint of blurred vision and pounding headache, is that right?" If this had happened to you in real life you would have probably nodded your head slowly, secretly hoping you made the right decision agreeing with the rest of what he said. If this scenario sounds familiar, you are not alone. Remember, 40-90 million Americans have difficulty understanding what the doctor says.

When You Don't Understand What the Doctor Says

Patients and their families-not doctors- are responsible for managing medical conditions outside of the hospital setting. This statement may catch you a bit off guard and yet it is true. Let's take for example the treatment of diabetes. Diet, exercise, stress reduction, and self-monitoring are the cornerstones of diabetic care. It is the diabetic who has to do the exercise, prepare his meals, monitor his blood sugars, and manage his or her stress. Without adequate knowledge of how do these things, the patient will not be able prevent the complications associated with poorly-controlled diabetes. Patients with poorly-controlled diabetes are more likely to have nerve pain, kidney failure, amputations, blindness, and stroke. Most patients, regardless of their disease process, who do not understand how to care for themselves will have more complications and suffer worse outcomes than patients who do understand and are able to follow their treatment plans.

In addition to having worse outcomes overall, patients with lower healthcare literacy are more likely to make expensive emergency room visits and to undergo unnecessary tests and procedures, all of which increase their chances of becoming a victim of a medical error. The Institute for Healthcare Advancement estimates healthcare costs for people with low healthcare literacy to be four times greater than for those with higher levels of literacy. When you are able to openly exchange information with your doctor and others, the quality of care you receive increases and your risk of suffering hurt and harm because of medical error decreases. That's why you need to understand what your doctor says and to be in charge of your healthcare.

CHAPTER THREE

Understanding What Your Doctor Just Said

"The safety of patients cannot be assured without mitigating the negative effects of low health literacy and ineffective communications on patient care."

The Joint Commission

How Your Culture Influences Communication With Your Doctor

Culture is the sum total of how a group of people live. It builds up over time and is transmitted from one generation to another. Culture includes the traditions of food, music, art, religion, and healthcare practices. It also dictates how members of a group communicate with one another and with their authority figures and doctors are revered authority figures in most cultures.

While cultural responses are rich in tradition, they

may prevent patients from speaking up and giving their doctors enough information to make the right diagnosis. For example, an older Chinese woman would probably be quite uncomfortable challenging her doctor's opinions, even if she completely disagreed them. In Asian cultures, authority figures are not questioned or challenged. A proper cultural response for her would be to show respect and gratitude for the information she had been given and to politely thank the doctor for his time and the services he rendered. Being submissive and not informing the doctor that he misunderstood what she was saying could be a problem if the doctor based his treatment plan upon that misunderstanding.

In the next few pages I have summarized the healthcare communication styles of European, African, Latin, and Asian Americans. This information does not include the nuances of every group or of each individual within these groups, as that would be impossible to do in this book. Instead, I have tried to give you a sense of the most common communication styles within each of the larger groups. I have done so because it is important that each of us understand how our culture affects our style of communication and how our style of communication affects our healthcare outcomes.

European Americans

Many European Americans have greater than average healthcare literacy. They also have the best healthcare outcomes in our nation. This group shows a willingness to research and learn about their conditions and to share that information with their doctors. In short, they are the group most likely to take an active role in the healthcare decision making process.

European Americans tend to equate health with mental and physical well-being. Their healthcare practices are based on a "scientific" approach and things research can prove. The scientific/research model includes the belief that it is possible to master one's health through scientific evaluation, periodic physical exams, laboratory testing, avoiding harmful substances, and performing activities that improve ones health such as exercise, proper diet, and stress reduction.

Among European cultures, it is accepted that the doctor uses a specialized language that the patient may not understand. They trust the doctor will explain any unknown concepts to them. A 2007 Veterans Affairs study, which reviewed trends in healthcare disparities, supports this notion. In the study, doctors gave European patients more information and counseling than their African American counterparts. As a result, the European Americans in the study had better understanding of their treatment options and what would happen during their time in the healthcare system, and they were more likely to undergo curative treatments.

On the other hand, older European Americans, those who are very sick, those with lower levels of healthcare literacy are just as vulnerable to medical error as members of any other cultural group. Other factors that negatively affect communication between Europeans and their doctors are:

- Very high trust levels in doctors, which may lead to "handing over" the decision making process to the doctor.

- High levels of trust in the scientific method which may lead to the overuse of medications and invasive procedures, both of which can have dangerous side effects.

African Americans

African Americans place a greater emphasis on the natural and spiritual aspects of health and have less reverence for the scientific model than their European counterparts. As a result, African Americans are less likely to study and or research conventional medical treatment and as a result they are less likely to be as proactive or to speak up for themselves in health matters. In the 2007 Department of Veterans Affairs study of healthcare disparities, hundreds of doctor/patient visits were evaluated for factors that could explain why European American have better healthcare outcomes than do African Americans. The researchers found that African Americans tended to passively accept the recommendations of their doctors; they gave less information, and asked fewer questions than their white counterparts.

This being said, effective communication is a two-way street. Healthcare literacy is not only a matter of how well the patient speaks and understands the language of medicine, it is also about how well the doctor speaks with the patient. Doctors in the study gave African Americans less information about the risks and benefits of procedures that could have easily helped them. Consequently, the patients in the study were more reluctant to undergo potentially curative procedures than were their European American counterparts. Overall, the study found African Americans receive less counseling, fewer up-to-date therapies, and inferior healthcare when being treated by the same providers with the same insurance coverage.

Another factor that influences the communication process between African Americans and their doctors is that the two groups have different styles of communication. For many African Americans, story telling is a major form of communication. Doctors, on the other hand, tend to communicate in a very direct manner and want to get directly to the point. Vital information can be lost if the patient begins telling a story about his or her illness and the doctor either cannot decipher the cultural meanings of the story or if he becomes impatient and stops listening the story. In summary, the following cultural and communications issues affect the quality of care African Americans receive:

- African Americans tend to have a low level of healthcare literacy.

- Patients are given less education by their healthcare providers

- Differences in communication styles may lead to patients being misunderstood and/or ignored.

Hispanics

Hispanics come from many countries around the world. They share the Spanish language and many beliefs about health. Many Hispanics believe health is a gift from God and a sign of good luck. They believe illness is punishment from God for wrongdoing, and that it can be prevented or relieved by repenting, praying, wearing religious symbols, and by atoning for one's sins. Some Hispanics will seek the help of a priest or a local healer before seeking the help of a doctor. When Hispanics do enter the healthcare system, they tend to believe the doctor is to be obeyed and that questioning him is impolite.

Language is also a tremendous barrier to Hispanics receiving quality healthcare. Many inner-city Hispanics have less than a high school education and are unable to read or write in either Spanish or English. It has been reported that 20 percent of Hispanics avoid going to the doctor because they cannot speak English. An inability to understand English and basic healthcare instructions greatly increases this groups' chances of falling victim to medical error. In summary, some of the cultural communication issues that negatively affect the healthcare outcomes of Hispanics are:

- Lower than average literacy and healthcare literacy, making it difficult to understand educational materials.

- A cultural belief that it is impolite to question the doctor or his authority.

- Overall language barriers.

Asians

Members of many Asian cultures believe physical health is determined by the quality of ones life force energy, called Chi or Prana. This energy is the essence of life and health. Yin and yang represent the opposite sides of the life force energy, equating to male and female, hot and cold, activity and rest, and so on. When the yin and yang components are properly balanced, the person is healthy and happy.

When communicating with doctors, Asians tend to be very respectful and polite. It is considered rude among older members of this group to ask questions; instead they may smile and nod even if they do not understand what is being said and to accept treatments that are given without question.

Even when asked for their opinions, many Asians will not openly state them out of "respect" for the doctor.

Outward expression of pain or emotion for many Asians is unacceptable. Often the only indication that there is a problem in an Asian patient is facial grimacing, silent withdrawal during tests or procedures, or an untouched food tray. It is also culturally correct for family members to keep "bad" news from the patient, because it is thought that upsetting the patient weakens the life force energy and robs the patient the power needed to recover from illness.

While all of the above are noble traditions, they can lead to ineffective or harmful treatments while delaying more appropriate care. In summary, the following cultural traditions may affect communication and the care an Asian Americans receive while in the healthcare system:

- Low conventional healthcare literacy

- Cultural barriers to asking questions

- Cultural barriers to voicing complaints

- Reluctance to reveal when they do not understand what is being said

- Cultural barriers to giving sick patients fully-informed consent

How Your Culture Affects Your Overall Treatment Plan

If your mother gave you a special tonic or tea when you were sick and you and your family members got better with those treatments, you will probably prefer to try your cultural medicines before trying medication from the pharmacy. If your culture discourages the use of medications or if you were taught a basic distrust of the medical system (like many African American are) you will not be inclined to follow the recommendations of a doctor who prescribes medication and surgery on the first visit. Formulating a treatment plan you understand and are willing to follow depends on your level of healthcare literacy; the relationship you have with the doctor who prescribed the treatment; how well the plan is communicated to you; and how well the plan fits into your cultural beliefs about health and healthcare.

Later in this chapter, you will learn how to talk with your doctors using O.L.D.C.A.R.T.S.—the standardized format doctors use to talk with you. You will learn to speak in a way that will gain you the attention and respect of your providers, and thereby affect all of your healthcare decisions, regardless of you your cultural style of communication.

Before we begin that process, you will need to learn how to gather and understand the information you want to share with your doctor during the visit. In other words, we are about to begin increasing your healthcare literacy and developing the skill sets you need to be the leader of **YOUR** Healthcare Team. Let's get started.

How To Increase Your Healthcare (Communication Skills) Literacy

To make any real changes in our lives, we must first commit to those changes. So, here and now I am asking you to commit to protecting the health and safety of you and your loved ones; to commit to increasing your healthcare knowledge and literacy; and to commit to becoming the leader of **YOUR** Healthcare Team and to begin that process by following the steps below.

Your role as team leader:
Don't be ashamed of what you don't know. Often, patients will hide the fact they do not understand what the doctor is saying because they are ashamed or embarrassed by their lack of understanding. Don't be! Most of you reading this book do not have medical degrees, and there is no reason to feel you should understand everything a doctor says.

Say "I don't understand." If there is anything you don't understand say, "I don't understand. Could you explain that to me?" If the doctor uses medical terms, you may want to say, "Could you explain that to me in plain English, please?" Often, doctors don't realize they're speaking in their own language (which is medical Latin). You may need to remind your doctor that he is speaking Latin and ask him to speak in plain English so that you can understand what he is saying.

When a doctor explains what he is saying in a language you can understand, it is more than a courtesy to you. Doctors have a legal obligation to teach you about your illnesses, the treatments you need, alternatives to those treatments, and about any risks you face while undergoing those treatments. Together, all of those things equate to giving the patient informed consent, which is required by law. If you are not given informed consent your doctor has not met his legal, ethical or moral obligations to you.

Use the Internet to gain more information even if you do not own a computer. Before I begin this section, I would like to say a few words about the Internet. First, if you do not have a computer, that's okay. Many local libraries have computers set up for residents of their municipalities to use. In addition, most teaching hospitals have libraries that are available for health-related research and are open to the family members of patients in the hospital.

If you have never used the Internet, don't worry. It's not difficult; the hardest part is learning how to click a button.

Librarians at either public or hospital libraries can show you what to do and you'll be "surfing the web" in no time flat.

If you are a beginning researcher, I suggest you rely heavily on the sites I recommend because they are well known and have a great deal of credibility. Believe it or not, not everything you'll read on the Internet is true. To judge a site, first make sure the person who authored the site is reputable, has solid credentials, and that he or she is not a quack selling tonic out of the back of their car. If you are reading about a drug, you will want to double check the information you find on sites owned by the drug's manufacturer because you may not get the whole truth on a commercial site. Use your common sense, be a critical-thinker, be careful, learn a lot, and have fun.

Once on the Internet, you will have access to symptom checkers that can help you and the doctor find the right diagnosis; you will be able to research the most up-to-date treatment guidelines; and learn how to safely take your medications. I address the use of each of those topics below.

Symptom checkers. Symptom checkers are tools into which you type a list of symptoms and they deliver to you the names of all the conditions in thier database that match your symptoms. Symptom checkers were created because there are thousands of human illnesses and no one can know all of them. A missed diagnosis can occur simply because the doctor may have either forgotten about the condition or because they never learned about the condition you have. Symptom checkers help ensure that no potential diagnosis is overlooked. They are not meant to, and should not claim to, diagnose your disease. The intended purposes of symptom checkers are to:

- Help ensure you have the right diagnosis,

- Help you to gather a list of possible diagnosis to discuss with your doctor, and to

- Help you develop a list of questions to ask your doctor, before you go into the office.

I like the symptom checkers listed below because they are located on very reputable sites; they are easy to use; and the information they provide is written for the non-medical person, so it's very easy to understand.

- www.WebMD.com

- www.About.com

- www.Mayoclinic.com

Research the latest treatment guidelines. The National Guideline Clearinghouse at www.guideline.gov is a comprehensive database of treatment guidelines written by the top medical experts in the country. The site's goal is to provide access for patients and providers to the most up-to-date treatment recommendations. After you are given a diagnosis, you can compare the experts' recommendations with the treatment your doctor has prescribed for you. After reading the information provided on the site you will be able to ensure you are getting the best care possible, and you will have enough information to discuss any discrepancies between what the experts recommend and what your provider has suggested to you do.

The consensus guidelines, for the most part, contain conventional treatments (treatments that are likely to be prescribed in the doctor's office). The guidelines may or may not include diet, nutritional supplements, exercise, education, natural and alternative therapies, or support group information.

The information on the sites listed below include information that will help you develop a comprehensive and wholistic care plan when combined with the medical recommendations found at www.guideline.gov and those prescribed by your doctor. Some of the sites you may want to look at are:

- www.WebMD.com

- www.Ask.com

- www.Mayoclinic.com

- www.AHRQ.gov (This site features disease-specific questions for many illnesses you may want to ask your doctor.)

- Sites that represent a condition or a disease, such as the American Heart Association or the American Cancer Society will have information that is helpful for managing the diseases they represent.

Research medication side effects and interactions. More than 7,000 patients die every year because of medications prescribed by doctors. By doing a bit of research, you can learn to how to take your medications safely and prevent many common medication errors. When you share what you have learned with your doctor, you will help her to safely prescribe your medications to you. I like the following sites for medication information:

- www.Drugs.com

- www.Walgreens.com

- www.Riteaid.com

- www.Medlineplus.gov

- www.WebMD.com

- www.Mayoclinic.com

Watch health segments on television. Watching health segments on television is another way to increase your knowledge and understanding of the latest medical research findings, medications, diet, and exercise trends. When you watch health segments on television, you have free access to experts on any number of health topics. Enjoy the show!

Read books and magazine articles. Health articles in your favorite magazines are informative, easy-to-read, and consumer-friendly sources of knowledge about healthcare issues. They are often written by medical professionals who are experts in their field and have a wealth of knowledge to share with their patients. I like to read these articles while I wait on the checkout line at the grocery store. I learn a lot and it passes the time.

Attend a class or workshop. Classes at your local hospital or community center are a great way to access local experts. Many experts teach small groups of patients about issues like as high blood pressure, diabetes, stroke, home care issues, and more. These classes are usually presented at little or no cost. Check the Websites of the your area hospitals for a list of their educational offerings.

Attend a support group meeting. Support groups are excellent sources of information and social support. Group members typically share similar experiences; they help each other to understand the choices they have to make; and what to expect while being treated for their condition. Research has shown that women who attend breast cancer support groups live longer than women who do not. Get out to a support meeting, make a friend, find support, increase your knowledge, feel better, and live longer!

Get in touch with your culture and how it affects your healthcare preferences. Once you have researched your condition and learned about your treatment options, you will be able to decide which options align with you and your cultural preferences. Maybe you believe in prayer as a treatment. Do you believe in the healing power of herbs and teas? These and many other therapies are rooted in native cultures from around the world and are used by more than one-third of Americans.

Be sure to research your natural therapy choices too. It is a good idea to print out the information you have gathered and take it with you to the doctor's office so that she can review the information for herself. This type of exchange will create and promote an interactive relationship in which both team members, you and the doctor, have something to contribute. This is what teamwork is all about.

When your doctors know more about your natural therapies, they will be better able to counsel you about how they will affect your conventional medicine care plan. And, your doctors enhanced knowledge about natural therapies increases the probability of you and your doctor being able to develop a treatment plan that aligns with your cultural beliefs.

After you have read about and explored issues concerning your care, you will be able to confidently communicate with your doctors. And, your doctors will be better able to communicate with you because the two of you will share a common knowledge base and a common language.

You will also know a good deal about your condition(s) and will be able to understand what the doctor is saying. You will no longer be subject to blindly following instructions with which you do not agree because you don't know what else to do. You and your provider will be able to make choices that align with your beliefs, your culture, and what you want for your life. Healthcare literacy is a very powerful tool in the pursuit of and receiving high quality healthcare.

Help Your Doctor Understand What You Just Said

After you have learned about your illnesses, medications, and treatment options you are almost ready to have a conversation about what you have learned with your doctor. However, there may still be two significant barriers to that conversation. As we have discussed, the first barrier is that the doctor speaks medical Latin and you speak your native language. Unless you are a medical professional, those are two different languages. The second barrier is that doctors are very busy people who think and speak very rapidly. Research shows that on average it takes a doctor approximately eighteen seconds from the time you begin talking before he begins to form a tentative diagnosis. This means you have about eighteen seconds to tell your story in a way you can be heard, understood, and given a proper diagnosis.

The average person has no idea how to tell the story of an illness he or she has had for several weeks in eighteen seconds without leaving out important details. Patients tend to want to tell the whole story of their illness, even if that illness that has been going on for years. Most doctors will not have the time or the patience to listen to a story that starts in 2000 and includes every detail of what has happened since then.

To enable you to speak with providers in the most efficient and concise way, I am going to teach you a communication technique called O.L.D.C.A.R.T.S. O.L.D.C.A.R.T.S (or some variation of it) is a primary language tool for healthcare providers of every discipline. It allows the provider to organize what you say to them in a format that highlights the information needed to make a diagnosis. O.L.D.C.A.R.T.S is a very good tool, but it is not perfect because any information you give the provider that does not fit into the O.L.D.C.A.R.T.S format may be discarded.

O.L.D.C.A.R.T.S is an acronym for *onset, location, duration, characteristics, associated and aggravating factors, relieving factors, timing, and severity.* If you have ever been to the doctor's office or an emergency room, you are familiar with answering questions in an O.L.D.C.A.R.T.S format. See if the following example sounds familiar to you:

> *"Good morning, Mrs. Jones. When did your stomachache start?"*
>
> *"Mrs. Jones, can you point to where it hurts?"*
>
> *"What does the pain feel like? Is it sharp or dull, does it come and go, or is it constant?"*
>
> *"Are you able to eat?"*
>
> *"How long after you eat does the pain start?"*
>
> *"Is there any nausea or vomiting, any constipation or diarrhea, fever, chills?"*
>
> *"What makes it worse? Spicy foods, milk, meat, fried foods?"*
>
> *"What makes it better? Antacids, rest?"*
>
> *"On a scale of 1-10 how bad is the pain?"*
>
> *"Are your symptoms triggered by stress?"*

O.L.D.C.A.R.T.S Sample Questions and Their Meanings

Question	Meaning
When did your stomachache start?	Onset
Can you point to where it hurts?	Location
How long does the pain last?	Duration
Is it sharp or dull? Does it come and go? Or is it constant?	Characteristics
Do you have any nausea or vomiting? Any constipation or diarrhea? Fever or chills?	Associated symptoms
What makes it worse? Spicy foods, milk, meat, fried foods, stress?	Aggravating factors
What makes it better?	Relieving factor
Is there any special time the pain comes on or goes away? How long after you eat does the pain occur?	Timing
On a scale of one to ten, how bad is the pain? How have the symptoms made you change your life?	Severity

Now that you have read these sample questions asked in the O.L.D.C.A.R.T.S format, you realize you have been asked questions in this format every time you've seen a healthcare provider. After the provider asks his questions, he will be listening for answers in this format as well.

Let's look at how Mrs. Jones answers the questions. In the first example, she answers the way many patients would. In a second example, we will learn how to answer the questions in the O.L.D.C.A.R.T.S format.

Mrs. Jones, replies, *"Well doctor, I'm not exactly sure when the pain started it may have been when I ate the food I left on the stove a few nights ago, but it may have been after the cookout at my sister's house last month. I ate a lot of food there. It was all so good. But I'm not sure if it was the same thing or not, because the pain at my sister's house came on and stayed for two days, but this pain was real sharp and it came and went and then it came back an hour later after I…."*

While Mrs. Jones' answer is not wrong, it is confusing. At the end of the story the doctor is still not sure when the pain started—was it month ago or was it last night? Was it from eating a combination of foods or was it from eating spoiled food? Is this a recurring problem or two separate problems? These are all questions the doctor is left with after this answer and this is only the first question. If your doctor begins to feel impatient during your story, it is likely he will cut you off in the middle of your story and rush you to a conclusion. In that rush important details of your story may be left out.

Now let's look at what happens when Mrs. Jones answers the questions about her stomachache in the O.L.D.C.A.R.T.S format.

Mrs. Jones: *"The pain started two nights ago. I ate food that had been left on the stove for about 36 hours and began having stomach cramps that were pretty constant and very painful six hours later. Then, I had eight very loose and watery stools over a 24-hour period. I did not have a fever or vomiting. I was not able to work because of the pain in my stomach was an 8-10 on the pain scale."*

In the first answer Mrs. Jones gave, it is clear she had not really thought about the answers to the questions the doctor would ask and as result she rambled on without clear direction. In the second example, when she answered the questions using the O.L.D.C.A.R.T.S format, she was clear and concise. She had thought about her answers and was prepared to get an accurate diagnosis and treatment plan. She also gave her doctor a good deal of information in a very short period of time. Thus, she freed up valuable time for further exploration, conversation, and education.

Speaking in an O.L.D.C.A.R.T.S format requires preparation, forethought, and self-examination before going to the doctor's office. The good news is that after reading this section of the book you will know what questions need to be answered well in advance of the visit, and you will have time to prepare your answers. The time you spend preparing the presentation of symptoms is well worth the effort.

In addition to all of the benefits already mentioned, this type of communication will promote trust and confidence in your doctor. When you are sure your doctor has heard you and understands your problems, you will be able to trust his opinions. When you trust that your doctor's opinions are accurate, you are more likely to carefully follow the treatment plans upon which the two of you agree. That means you will get better care.

Below are the questions to think about and answer before going to the doctor's office. In conjunction with the O.L.D.C.A.R.T.S. questions on the following pages, I have given you the type of information that should be included in your answers. In the Appendix you will find an O.L.D.C.A.R.T.S worksheet on which you can write your answers. After you have completed the worksheet, practice telling your story so that you can deliver it in a clear and organized fashion. Take the completed worksheet with you to the visit to help you remember dates, times, and important details.

The O.L.D.C.A.R.T.S. Worksheet

• **Onset**

When did the problem begin? Was it after you ate? Did you hurt yourself? Did anything trigger your symptoms? Was the onset slow or was it rapid? Were you exposed to any new foods or chemicals? Were you upset or angry? Are you going through a stressful time (job loss, divorce, problems with your children)?

• **Location of the problem**

Where is the problem? In addition to naming the part of your body that is affected, it is a good idea to physically point to the area on your body. This will help avoid confusion and ensure you and the doctor are talking about the same thing. To a provider, the stomach is located in the arch of the rib cage. A patient may believe the stomach is in the area of the naval. To avoid confusion, always point to the area of your body that is hurting and to the other parts of your body that are affected by your problem.

• **Duration**

Duration includes two dimensions: how long do the symptoms last once they start (such as one hour, all day, they never stop) and how long the condition itself has been going on (such as one week, two months, or a year). Think about and answer both parts of the question.

- **Characteristics**

Pain and other symptoms have characteristics that are best explained using descriptive words. Use words that produce feelings and images to which the doctor can relate, such as stabbing pain, crushing pain, or sharp pain. These are descriptive words that are often used to describe sensations in the body, and they help the provider identify what part of the body is being affected by your problem. For example, sensations of numbness and tingling are generally associated with a nerve condition. Colicky pain indicates the problem is in a hollow organ like the stomach. Think carefully about your symptoms and their characteristics because they will give your providers important clues and help them to formulate an accurate diagnosis.

- **Associated Symptoms**

What symptoms accompany your primary complaint (the thing that is bothering you the most and brought you to the doctor's office)? If you have a stomachache, do you also have fever, chills, nausea, vomiting, or diarrhea? Do you have an appetite? Are you able to eat as much as you used to? If you cannot eat, how long has it been since you have eaten? What would happen if you try to eat now? If you have vomiting or diarrhea describe how much, how often, and what it looks like. I know this is not the most pleasant of topics; however, all of this information is important and it gives your provider clues that will help him make the right diagnosis and prescribe the best treatment plan.

Report all associated factors, even if no one asks you about them. Do not think that if the doctor didn't ask, it must not be important. Doctors cannot and do not remember to ask everything. It is quite possible that he or she may forget to ask a question that would give them much-needed information. Volunteer information freely because it may be important for the provider to know.

- **Aggravating Symptoms**

This questions asks, what makes your condition worse? Does your back hurt more when you sleep on a soft mattress or when you lift heavy objects? Does your stomach hurt more when you eat spicy or fried foods? If so, these are aggravating factors.

- **Relieving Factors/Treatments Tried**

Relieving factors are things that make you feel better. Do your symptoms improve when you move, eat, drink, take an over-the-counter medication, or eat Grandma's chicken soup? Does heat or sleep make you to feel better? If so, these are relieving factors. Report anything that makes your symptoms better. Report how much relief you get from your treatments and how long the relief lasts before the symptoms return. You should also report all the treatments you have tried and whether they did or did not relieve the problem. Reporting all treatments tried will save valuable time by helping the doctor avoid prescribing treatments that haven't worked in the past. He or she can then focus on treatments that have helped you or suggest something new.

- **Timing**

Timing asks the questions when do your symptoms occur and in relationship to what? Do you become dizzy when you stand up? Do you get heartburn 20 minutes after you eat or two hours after you eat? Do your symptoms start in the morning upon rising? Do they start after an argument with your spouse? Or, did they begin after you started a new prescription or over-the-counter medication? How long did they begin after you started the new medication?

A word to the wise, always consider drug side effects and drug-to-drug interactions as the source of any new problem without a clear cause. If a healthcare provider misses the fact that your new symptoms are actually side effects of a medication, you may get a new diagnosis and even more medications to treat your side effects. This can become a vicious cycle; one in which you will not get better. Always consider medication side effects as a possible cause of your problems!

- **Severity**

Severity asks how strong your symptoms are and how much your symptoms have caused you to change your life. Regarding pain, you will probably be asked how severe the pain is on a scale of 1-10. Is your pain a minor annoyance (a 1-2 on the pain scale) or do you have mild to moderate discomfort (2-4)? Are you really uncomfortable (a 5-6 on the pain scale) and feel you need to take something to relieve the pain? Or is the pain severe (7- 9) and making your life miserable? If the pain is an excruciating (10 or above), you *must* seek help.

When reporting pain and discomfort, you also want to report how the symptoms have changed your life. Does your stomach hurt so much you have not been able to eat for five days? Does your head hurt so badly you cannot tolerate sound or light? Is the muscle weakness to the point where you can no longer open a jar or hold your cell phone? Understanding the full impact your illness has on your life brings deeper meaning to your pain and suffering because it becomes more than a number on a scale. It is very important that the provider "feel" for you because this helps her to act in caring ways and motivates her to bring you relief.

When asked what they want in a doctor, patients often respond that they want someone they can talk to, someone who will listen to them, and someone who understands and has compassion for their situation. These types of caring relationships are based on effective communication and mutual respect. Speaking in the O.L.D.C.A.R.T.S format will help you and your provider develop this type of relationship by improving the quality of your communication and thereby improving your level of healthcare safety.

CHAPTER FOUR

How to Choose the Right Doctor and Get Better Care

"The good physician treats the disease; the great physician treats the patient who has the disease."

William Osler M.D.

Looking For Dr. Right

Choosing a doctor is one of the most important decisions you will ever make. Quite literally, your life could depend upon your choice(s). If your doctor treats your condition improperly, you could be injured or killed by the care you receive. Prior to making a choice of such magnitude, it is important to decide what it is you want. When you know what you want, you are better prepared to search for and find the object of your desire.

In a 1992 survey conducted by a Dr. Delbanco, patients

were asked what they wanted in a doctor. The patients said they wanted:

- Doctors who are competent and know how to do their jobs well

- Doctors who will treat them with dignity and respect

- The ability to negotiate effectively with the doctor

- A doctor who will explain how their sickness and treatments will affect their lives.

- A doctor who will be honest and tell them what they want and need to know.

- Someone who will teach them how to care for themselves away from the clinical setting

- A doctor who will focus on pain, discomfort, and disabilities and a

- A doctor who is sensitive to their individual and cultural needs.

If you have a doctor who has all of those characteristics, you have found Dr. Right, and unless you are looking for a specialist or a second opinion, you do not need to finish reading this chapter. If you have not found Dr. Right, some work may be required to find him because it is not wise to select someone who plays such a critical role on *YOUR* Healthcare Team by simply looking through the phone book.

Before you begin the selection process, there is a concept I want you to clearly understand, and that concept is this: You are the owner of *YOUR* Healthcare Team and your doctors are your employees, they work for you and they make their living by collecting your insurance dollars. There is no doubt that your doctors are very important employees; nonetheless they are employees. You must be clear that your doctors work for you, otherwise you will believe they are in charge of your healthcare, and you will not be empowered to make choices based on your wants and needs. Instead, you may be inclined to accept whoever and whatever care they deliver and that's not the best thing for you or your loved ones.

When choosing a doctor, you will need to evaluate the candidates for the position in three essential categories: accessibility, skill level, and personality (bedside manner). To start the selection process, you will first need to review your insurance carrier's list of providers and the narrow down that list to providers to those who meet your specific needs.

With a list of candidates in hand, ask your other doctors, your family members, and friends if they either recommend or discourage the use of any doctors on your list. If you know any nurses who work at your area hospitals, ask them who they would recommend. Nurses know the best and worst doctors because they have worked with many of them over time and in a variety of situations. Nurses know which doctors are competent, kind, and trustworthy, all qualities you want in a doctor, and they know the doctors who do not possess those qualities as well.

Your next step is to evaluate each candidate's credentials and their safety records. Several reputable Internet sites can help you to verify a provider's training, specialty certifications, and any disciplinary actions that may have been leveled against the doctor. Currently, HealthGrades.com is the most comprehensive resource for examining a doctor's background in all of these areas. The American Medical Association also collects safety information on its members, and a handful of states gather and report malpractice information. Other Internet sites where you can investigate a doctor's qualifications and malpractice records are:

- www.RateMD.com (includes patient feedback on doctors)

- www.physicianreports.com

- To find out if your state makes malpractice information available to the public, call your local Board of Health.

The following two sets of questions will help you evaluate a doctor in terms of training, skills, accessibility, and beside manner. Many of the questions on the first worksheet can be answered by the office staff or by researching the provider on the Internet.

Questions to Ask When Choosing a Doctor

• **Is the provider part of your insurance plan?**

Generally speaking, if the answer to this question is "no" your plan will not pay for the care rendered unless your plan allows you to use out-of-network providers. If you do not have out-of-network benefits, but need to see an out-of-network provider because he or she has specialty training, contact your insurance plans' case manager and explain your circumstances. The case manager may be able to get you the care you need by negotiating a contract with the doctor whose expertise you need. You may incur extra costs; however, if you need the care *only* this doctor can provide, it may be well worth it.

• **Does the clinician have the background and training you need?**

In general, everyone needs a general practitioner or internist to manage their colds and flu and their minor aches and pains. For more serious problems, you many need to see a specialist. Specialists have more training and knowledge in their area of study than do general practitioners, who specialize in treating everything. If you have an uncontrolled disorder or a newly-diagnosed condition, you may want to ask your internist for a referral to a specialist.

- **Is the doctor board certified?**

Board certified it means the doctor has completed extra hours of clinical training and has passed a national certification examination that has earned him or her the title "board certified." Lack of board certification does not mean the provider is not qualified to care for you. It simply means the doctor has not completed the board certification process. When searching for a specialist, you probably want to eliminate providers who are not board certified and have not completed specialty training.

- **Is there a long wait to get an appointment?**

If you have a condition for which you need immediate attention such as a new diagnosis of cancer, out-of-control blood sugar, or really high blood pressure, you need to be seen as soon as possible. In such cases, long waits to get an appointment are not acceptable or safe. Consider removing a provider who has really long waits from your list of candidates.

- **How long is the wait in the waiting room?**

Sometimes things happen, and you may experience a longer than usual wait in the waiting room. However, if long waits are the norm in the office this may not be what you need, especially if you are not feeling well, have special equipment, or need someone to accompany you to the visit as your advocate will have to wait too, and you will want to be mindful of your advocates' time as well. Ask the office staff and others in the waiting room about the average wait time and make a decision.

- **How much time is scheduled for appointments?**

When you call to make an appointment, ask the receptionist how much time is scheduled for each appointment. At a bear minimum, fifteen minutes should be allotted for appointments, more time is better than less time.

- **Which hospital does the doctor use and do you want to go to that hospital? Is the hospital in your health plan?**

There is always the risk you will be hospitalized, and where you are hospitalized makes a difference. Some hospitals are better than others. If the potential provider is on staff at the best hospital in your area and your health plan covers care at that facility, wonderful. If the doctor is only on staff at the worst hospital in the area, (read more about this in Chapter Twelve), and you are not comfortable going to that hospital, this may not be the doctor for you.

- **Does the doctor care for hospitalized patients?**

Some doctors do not care for hospitalized patients. Those doctors use the services of a hospitalist to care for their hospitalized patients. A hospitalist is a physician on staff at the hospital who cares for patients in emergencies and when the patient does not have an attending/private physician. If it is important to you that you are cared for by your doctor when you are in the hospital, you will want to know if the doctor provides that service or if he visits surrenders the care of his hospitalized patients to a hospitalist.

- **What are the office hours?**

Having evening hours is important if you or the friends and family members who will help with your care work during the day. Ask what the office hours are before signing up with a provider. Make sure the office hours fit your schedules.

- **Is the provider male or female?**

Does this matter to you? Do you want a male gynecologist

or a female urologist? Do you have religious restrictions that restrict you from having a male or female provider? Think this over and be honest with yourself. It may seem like a little thing, but if you ignore your preference and later find you are uncomfortable with your doctor's gender, this could interfere with communication between you and your doctor and that's is not a good thing. Make the choice that best fits your care needs and your comfort level.

- **Does the doctor's age matter to you?**

You may want a provider with whom you can grow old or one who is your own age and understands your lifestyle choices. You may want a provider who is up-and-coming or you may want an older, more experienced physician. It's your choice, but remember, it is a choice. If the doctor's age matters to you, ask the receptionist how old the doctor is before you make the appointment.

- **Is the doctor part of your native culture?**

Do you want a provider with whom you share the same culture? A doctor with your cultural background may be better able to help you make safe choices about using traditional medicines when combined with conventional medicines. He or she may also understand your beliefs and customs surrounding your care.

- **Does the doctor speak your native language?**

Communication is key, especially when making a diagnosis. If the doctor does not have a clear understanding of what you are saying, your chances of being misdiagnosed increase exponentially. If you find a provider who speaks your native language and meets the other employment criteria, he should be considered very strongly for the position of doctor on *YOUR* Healthcare Team.

- **Who covers for the provider when he she is not available? Does that person have the training needed to care for your special condition(s)?**

If you have multiple health problems, complicated care issues, or a special condition, you may need to see a specialist. If your doctor is a specialist, does she have a good team of associate doctors who are also qualified to take care of you when she is away. And don't forget to ask if the covering doctor speaks your language.

- **Does the doctor take phone calls from patients or give advice over the phone? Will the staff call in medication refills?**

Are you always able to go in to the office? Do you need help from someone else to go to the doctor? Do you travel a lot? If so, having the ability to get advice over the phone may be important to you. Having to go in to the office may also be challenging if you cannot afford the co-pay for an office visit every time you need is a prescription refilled.

Questions to Ask After the Office Visit

After meeting with the doctor, you will want to evaluate the doctors' bedside manner. This set of questions will help you to evaluate the doctor's communication skills; his ablility listen and to teach and his levels of respect, kindness and empathy toward you. The combination of these qualities equal the doctors bedside manner.

- **Did you feel comfortable talking with the doctor?**

If the answer to this question is "no" there may be no need to go any further. Teamwork and communication are essential to delivering safe patient care. You want to choose a provider you feel comfortable talking to.

- **Is the practitioner safe and knowledgeable?**

In addition to being properly trained, safe practitioners are well organized and in control of the information you need to know about your condition. Usually the advice a knowledgeable provider gives will match the information you found while researching your condition on the Internet. If the doctor is disorganized and unable to give you clear answers to your questions, you have met an unsafe provider. This is not the doctor for you.

- **Did the doctor respect your thoughts and opinions and encourage you to express them?**

No one knows better than you do what you are experiencing. If you feel something is wrong, your thoughts, perceptions, and experiences should be respected. If the doctor discounts what you say and indicates that your perceptions are wrong, she limits your ability to add to your healthcare safety. If a doctor dismisses your experiences she is not the doctor for you.

- **Did the practitioner spend enough time with you and give you her undivided attention? Or was she frequently interrupted?**

Interruptions equal mistakes. Practitioners need to be attentive to you. If the doctor is answering a pager, taking phone calls, or otherwise being interrupted during the visit (assuming this is her usual practice and not just a very busy day) this doctor is much too busy to give you the attention and safe care you deserve.

- **Did the provider answer your questions in terms you could understand?**

If a doctor does not answer questions in language you can understand, you should ask her to explain her answers in plain English. If after asking her to speak in plain English you still don't understand what the doctor said, this is probably not the doctor for you.

- **Did the doctor ask questions to ensure you understood his explanation?**

A good doctor knows you may not understand everything she says and will try to assess what you did and did not understand, by asking, "Do you understand and do you have any questions?"

- **Is the provider a good teacher?**

Did the provider teach you what you need to know about your condition? Did she teach you about diet, exercise, rest, and different types of therapy, or did she only discuss medications?

You are a whole person and your health depends on your overall well- being. A good doctor will give you a wholistic education.

- **Did the provider listen and allow you time to explain your problems without interrupting?**

Communication is just as much about listening as it is talking. A good provider will listen to you and attempt to understand you and your concerns.

- **Did the provider ask you what type of treatment you prefer?**

You are much more likely to follow a treatment plan you understand and with which you agree. A good doctor will take time to explain the risks and benefits of your treatment options and will not be threatened by your desire to explore options she did not suggest. The doctor should be able to discuss all of your options with to you in an open and fluid manner. She should then help you identify which option(s) will work best for you and why.

- **Did the provider wash his hands between patients?**

Hand washing is the single most important tool in preventing the spread of infection. If you do not notice a practitioner in any setting washing his hands between patients ask if they would mind doing so before beginning your exam. Asking may make you a bit uncomfortable, but it is better to be uncomfortable than to be infected with a serious disease.

After you have asked and answered these two sets of question you will be better able to choose the right doctor for *YOUR* Healthcare Team. Trust yourself and do not act hastily. You may want to go to several visits before making your final selection.

As a final note, when considering a primary care provider, please consider choosing a nurse practitioner. Nurse practitioners are very good primary care providers with a proven record of safety. In studies evaluating patient satisfaction with nurse practitioners, the patients reported being impressed with nurse practitioners in terms of their knowledge, communication style, accessibility, and bedside manner. Patients in the studies felt the nurse practitioners truly cared about them, and they were motivated to follow the nurse practitioner's instructions. Overall, the patients were very satisfied with the care they received from their nurse practitioners. This is a big decision think it over and choose wisely.

CHAPTER FIVE

When to Fire Your Doctor

"The mistakes made by doctors are innumerable."

Marcel Proust

Like any other person you hire to perform a service, your doctor may not work out, and you as the owner of **YOUR** Healthcare Team may need to fire your doctor. Your doctor holds a pivotal role on **YOUR** Healthcare Team, because his performance affects aspect of your care. You have a responsibility to yourself (and to those who love you) to terminate your doctor if he endangers your health or performs in ways you find unacceptable. In this chapter, I discuss situations in which the doctor should be let go from your team and situations when you and your doctor should talk with the hope that he will correct the unwanted behavior and the two of you will be able to go on together. Let's get started.

When the Doctor has to Go

When the doctor is incompetent. In some cases, there is no question the doctor is unsafe or incompetent and should be let go from your team. This is especially true when she has made a mistake that has hurt or endangered you. In other cases the doctor's incompetence may not be as easily discerned. Some of the behaviors that indicate you have an incompetent doctor are: he cannot remember the details of your case; he is not sure what the next steps should be; he has prescribed wrong and or unnecessary treatments; and/or he is disorganized and unprepared to give you proper care and counsel.

Your role as team leader:

- If you have evidence that your doctor is incompetent or if he has made a significant mistake in your case that cannot be explained or excused, fire your doctor.

- Seek a competent replacement.

The doctor does not listen to you or respect your thoughts and opinions. If your doctor does not respect your thoughts; cuts you off when you speak; walks away as you are talking; or dismisses your complaints and makes you question whether your symptoms are real or imagined; your doctor does not value your thoughts and opinions and he should be let go from *YOUR* Healthcare Team.

Dismissing your thoughts and feelings could lead to an inaccurate diagnosis. Studies have shown that patients are more accurate than doctors when diagnosising themselves with common ailments. Your thoughts and opinions are very important and they should be respected.

Your role as team leader:

- Ask the doctor not to dismiss your reports and to listen to you.

- Ask the doctor if he could look a little further for a diagnosis.

- Research your symptoms using a symptom checker. Take a printout of your findings with you to your doctor's office for review.

- If the doctor still does not respect your thoughts and opinions fire him and find someone who will.

The doctor does not communicate with you about your care plan. Maybe your doctor orders tests and does not tell you why, or gets test results and does not explain them to you. Or maybe he prescribes medications without telling you exactly what they are for; or maybe he doesn't return your calls and your questions seem to annoy him, you can safely assume your doctor is not communicating with you about your care plan in a way that will help you to receive safe and effective healthcare. It's time to look for another doctor.

Your role as team leader:

- Ask for detailed explanations of laboratory tests, diagnostic procedures, and their results.

- Ask why medications are being prescribed and how to take them safely.

- If the information is not forthcoming, fire your doctor and hire one who is willing to talk with you and answer your questions.

Your provider doesn't seem to care about you. When someone cares about you they want the best for you and are willing to think creatively to find solutions to your problems. If the doctor does not care, he will not be concerned with your needs and may even be outwardly cold toward you. If any of these situations sound familiar, it's time to fire your doctor and to find one who cares about you.

Having said that, there is a possible exception to this rule. If Dr. Coldhearted happens to be a surgeon and you trust she is the right person for the job, you may want to overlook her personality flaws. Because your relationship with a surgeon is usually short-term and the amount of kindness and empathy the doctor exhibits may not be as important as her ability to skillfully perform your surgery. On the other hand, if the surgeon is rude and doesn't listen to you, she could be a danger to your health and safety. You will have to weigh this for yourself.

Your role as team leader:

- When hiring a doctor, choose one who is kind and caring. Caring providers take time to listen and will do all that they can to ensure you receive the best care possible.

The doctor dehumanizes you. Dehumanization occurs when the doctor cares more about treatments and procedures than for you as a person. If the doctor doesn't seem to care how his treatments affected you and he is unresponsive to your needs, you are being dehumanized.

A Story About Being Dehumanized By Your Doctor

The day after surgery, your surgeon and his team of residents and interns come into your hospital room at five o'clock in the morning. They stand around your bed and discuss you as you lie there trying to figure out if the conversation you are hearing is real or a dream. At that very moment, your surgeon pulls back the bedcovers and rips the surgical dressing from your belly without warning. Now you know this is not a dream.

The young doctors gather around to observe the handiwork of their chief, each one peering over the head of the other, trying dutifully to observe your incision. After each one has had his or her turn looking at your wound, they all back away. The surgeon begins talking, and although he is talking *about* you, he is not talking *to* you. It's as if you aren't really in the room. You try to hear what the doctor is saying; however, you are only able to hear bits and pieces of what is said. The doctor rattles off a few things for the team to do today (order labs, get her out of bed, check the pathology report) and then, just as suddenly as they came, they all leave. They don't even say good-bye.

You lie there, cold, exposed, and vulnerable, your belly stinging in pain from the bandage being ripped away. You wonder what just happened. You wonder what your wound looks like. It would have been nice if they had talked to you about your incision or how you were feeling, your pain, your walking, your eating, your happiness, your sadness, or your discharge plan – anything at all about you would have been nice. However, it was not to be. When events like this happen, you have been dehumanized.

Your role as team leader:

- Tell the provider you would like time to express your concerns and to have your questions answered.

- If the doctor cannot or will not take time to talk with you, listen to your concerns, or to answer your questions, consider finding another doctor.

You cannot get an appointment. Waiting too long to get help could be dangerous. If you have pain, bleeding, or any other poorly controlled condition, waiting weeks for an appointment is unsafe and unacceptable.

Your role as team leader:

- Find a doctor with whom you can get an appointment in a timely fashion.

The doctor's office is really far away. If you are too sick to drive long distances and you have to make frequent trips to the doctor, it is best to have a provider who is near your home and uses ancillary services, such as labs and hospitals, that are close your home as well. Of course, this may not apply if you live in a rural area or if you need to see a specialist. Under these circumstances you must do whatever is necessary to get the care you need.

Your role as team leader:

- Whenever possible, choose a doctor who is located near your home. This will decrease the amount of time and money you spend on fuel and other travel expenses to see your doctor.

Things You Need to Discuss with Your Doctor

There are times when a doctor's behavior rises to the level of termination and you know he must be fired. There are other times when the doctors actions are not as damaging, and you may simply want to talk with him about your concerns. The following are some of the things your doctors may do that you need to discuss with him before his actions jeopordize your health and safety.

Doctors enter into contractual agreements with insurance companies that may not be in your best interest. Doctors enter into agreements with insurance companies whose terms have implications for the type of care you are offered. One published study found 35 percent of responding physicians reported they had not offered their patients treatments that may have helped them because of incentives to keep costs down or because of coverage restrictions.

Some of the contractual agreements doctors enter into have "gag rules" these are rules that prevent doctors from revealing whether they are paid to withhold treatment or to perform procedures. Under these same agreements there may be stipulations that prohibit the doctor from revealing treatments that have been withheld from you because of the type of insurance coverage you have. However, doctors are allowed to answer any and all of your questions about existing treatment options whether or not they are covered by your insurance plan.

Your role as team leader:

Research treatment options for your condition at:
- www. Guideline.gov

- www.WebMD.com

- www.Mayoclinic.com and other reputable sites.

- Compare your findings with what your doctor has recommended. If your doctor does not offer you treatments established by national guidelines or other credible sources, discuss the discrepancies with the doctor.

- If you believe reimbursement or insurance regulations are motivating the doctor's decisions, discuss your concerns with your provider. Tell him what you are thinking and ask if you are correct.

- If there is a test or procedure you need and your insurance company refuses to pay for it, contact the company's case manager and learn how to get approval for the procedure.

- If you can no longer trust your doctor or you feel he is more heavily motivated by insurance incentives than he is by caring for you and your well being, fire him.

The doctor is rude to other members of your team. If your doctor is mean or raises his voice to other team members, not only is this behavior unprofessional, immature, and totally unacceptable, it is also degrading to the person at whom the doctor is yelling. Being verbally abusive toward others is more than wrong and inappropriate; it is a barrier to you getting the best care possible, and it could create an unsafe situation for you.

When doctors are rude to other team members, I can assure you those team members will not be anxious to come running when you call. Instead they will want to avoid you and anything to do with you until they feel strong enough to withstand your doctor's attacks. Additionally, the stress of being publically humiliated upsets the attacked person and predisposes them to making even more mistakes.

Hurtful interactions also create communication barriers between team members who need to be able to talk and freely exchange information. The nurse is not going to go out of her way to call the doctor to report something he may need to know because she will have to speak to a rude and hurtful indiviual. When the two do speak, vital information may not be transmitted because verbally abusive language limits affective communication.

Your role as team leader:
- Do not condone or support rude, hurtful behavior toward other members of **YOUR** Healthcare Team.

- Let the doctor know you want him to control his outbursts, because they could get you into trouble.

- Tell the person who was hurt by the doctors' behavior that you do not condone the way the doctor behaved.

- Let other team members know you respect and value them, even if they have made a mistake. This will help decrease the team members' stress and make it less likely they will make another error. It also makes it more likely they will be willing to come when you call.

Sometimes doctors do not listen to other members of your health care team. When a doctor does not listen or makes it difficult for team members to express their opinions, things can go terribly wrong. Healthcare is a team effort, and all team members have something to contribute. If your doctor is an intimidator, your team members may not feel free to share information with the doctor or with you. This could create a problem for you down the road.

A Story About What Happens When Your Doctor Does Not Listen to Other Members of Your Team

One morning during rounds with Dr. Mean, Sue, a bright young resident, wanted to speak up and suggest that Mrs. Jones not be treated with a blood thinner. Mrs. Jones was at risk of having a massive bleed and the blood thinner greatly increased her risk. Sue didn't say anything because she felt Dr. Mean would not agree with her and she ran the risk of being publicly humiliated if she spoke up. The patient was given the blood thinner and ended up in ICU with a retroperitoneal hematoma (a huge blood clot in the back of the abdomen) that had to be surgically removed. Fortunately, the patient survived; however, that may not always be the case.

Your role as team leader:

- Know that many members of **YOUR** Healthcare Team (the physical therapist, the nutritionist, occupational therapist, and others) have years of training and valuable experience that may be helpful to you. (For example, a nutritionist with a Master's degree knows more about nutrition than a doctor who never took a class in nutrition, and a physical therapist who has earned a Ph.D. will know more about movement therapy than your general practitioner.)

- Take full advantage of your team members' specialty training by asking them to share their thoughts, opinions, and recommendations with you.

- Discuss the information you get from your team members with your doctors and decide if you would like to follow their suggestions.

- Let your doctor know you value the opinions of your other team members' and that you look forward to sharing the information you have gained.

Clearly, the doctor/patient relationship is a very important one. In order for it to work well there needs to be access to the provider; trust and respect between doctor and patient; and collaboration among team members. If these conditions do not exist because of barriers created by your doctor's behavior, fire your doctor. You can then hire one who has the skill set, training, expertise, and disposition you require of the top professional on *YOUR* Healthcare Team.

CHAPTER SIX

Choosing Personal and Professional Advocates

"We all need somebody to lean on."

Bill Withers

Why You Need an Advocate

Advocates are people who help protect the rights and beliefs of others. By definition, an advocate "helps another to plead his or her case." Anyone who enters the healthcare system may need someone to advocate for them because every aspect of the healthcare system can be challenging to negotiate. Just getting an appointment with a new doctor can be a confusing; to do so you must understand your insurance coverage; have access to a primary care provider; and be eligible to receive in- and out-of-network referrals. And this is just the beginning of the process. The challenges to accessing care go on and on, and they are even greater for the very sick, the elderly, and those who have difficulty understanding medical language. At some point any one of us may need an advocate to help navigate the healthcare maze or to help manage our illnesses.

Personal advocates give the patients they care for emotional, physical, and logistical support, and they can be invaluable assets to any healthcare team. The elderly parent, the disabled child, and the adult suffering from a debilitating disease might quite possibly perish without the help and support of an advocate/caregiver. In addition to helping and caring for their loved ones, many advocates arc also healthcare proxies (legal substitutes) for their loved ones. Your healthcare proxy and a living will are very important members of **YOUR** Healthcare Team. Let me explain why.

Should you become unable to speak for yourself, your healthcare proxy will speak for you. Your proxy bears the awesome responsibility of protecting your health and safety when you are completely vunerable and unable to protect yourself. Your living will, when properly completed, tells your proxy and other members of **YOUR** Healthcare Team what you would have said if you were able express you wishes. A living will relieves your proxy of the burden of having to make monumental decisions for you without your guidance.

It is of vital importance to your health and the well being of your loved ones that you appoint a healthcare proxy and complete a living will because the decisions made for you in a healthcare setting can and will affect the way you and your signifgant others spend the rest of your lives.

If for example the decision is made that you should be placed on a ventilator (a machine that breaths for you), you could live many years in a nursing home attached to that machine. Do you want that? Without input from you in the form of a living will, you may receive care you never wanted and your signifigant other could pay the price. Once a patient is placed in a nursing home, his or her assets (money) belong to both the nursing home and the spouse. Depending on your financial situation, you and your spouse could become bankrupt by the loss of part or all of your income as it will be paid to the nursing home. This cold, hard truth is reflected in the national statistic that tells us that every 30 minutes someone in America files for bankruptucy because of healthcare costs.

There are social and emotional issues that arise when families are suddenly thrust into making life-altering decisions without guidance from the injured party and a living will as well. Your family may be unable to decide upon a course of action and a bitter disagreement could develop; a disagreement that could tear your family apart. Family members experience a great deal of pain and agony when a loved one is seriously ill and they are forced to make life or death decisions without clear direction from the injured party, some of the suffering families experience during these times can be avoided by legally appointing a healthcare proxy and creating a living will.

A healthcare proxy is designated by the act of signing a medical power of attorney (POA). Once your POA is signed, notorized, and filed according to your state's regulations, it gives your proxy the authority to discuss your medical concerns with your healthcare providers and to make medical decisions, including those surrounding end-of-life care and terminating life support. (A medical power of attorney does not give your advocate the power to make legal or financial decisions. If you want to give your advocate or anyone else the power to make those decisions you will need a non-medical power of attorney.)

Now that you understand the importance of having a healthcare proxy and a living will, the questions become, "Who will be my healthcare proxy?" "What are my living will options and what will I choose?"

Choosing a Healthcare Proxy

Healthcare proxies are most commonly the patient's spouse, life partner, and children. Generally speaking, spouses are allowed to speak for one another without a medical POA; however, this privilege is not guaranteed. In cases of marital separation or if there is a history of abuse, and in situations where your family members or your caregivers disagree with your spouse, his or her decision may be successfully contested if your spouse is not your POA and you do not have a living will. The very best way to ensure the person you want to speak for you is allowed to do so is to complete a medical POA and to formally appoint that person to the position of healthcare proxy on **YOUR** Healthcare Team.

Whomever you choose should have the courage of your convictions and be willing to honor your wishes. If your daughter could not terminate your life support and you do not wish to be artificially sustained, she should not be your proxy. The person you choose should also have the strength to disagree with your daughter or anyone else who opposes your wishes, should the need arise. In addition to choosing someone who will honor and protect your wishes, you should choose:

- Someone who is dependable and will be there for you when you need help.

- Someone who will be available to talk with your doctors and go to appointments with you if necessary.

- Someone who is willing to spend time at your beside in the hospital where you will probably most need their help.

- Someone with good communication skills and gets along

well with others. (Arguing with other team members makes a really hard time a lot harder and can lead to receiving worse care.)

- Someone with a healthcare background (if possible) to help you understand and navigate the system.

Choosing one person to be your healthcare proxy can generate feelings of anger, jealousy, and rejection in those who were not chosen. To prevent negative emotions from flaring, the experts suggest having a family meeting to discuss your choice of proxy and your living will decisions with family members who would be involved in making decisions for you if you did not have a proxy and a living will. Anyone who is unable to attend the meeting should also be informed of your choices at some point.

A family meeting is more than a courtesy to your loved ones. It could help guarantee you get the kind of care you would like to have. If your spouse or any of your children objects to your wishes, he or she can contest your choices and prevent you from receiving the care you want until the dispute is resolved. Making your wishes known will encourage your family members to honor and respect your choices, even if they disagree with them.

At the family meeting it is important to tell your family members why you chose your advocate. Hopefully, those who were not chosen will understand and become comfortable with your decision after it is explained to them.

If you have more than one person you would like to be your advocate, you are a very fortunate person. You will, however, need to designate just one person. Having one person speak for you simplifies the communication process and helps to avoid the confusion and treatment delays that arise when doctors have to discuss treatment options and obtain consent from more than one person. Your second and third proxy choices can be named in your documents and designated to step in should your first choice become unable to perform his or her duties.

Living Wills and Their Options

A living will documents your wishes for care surrounding the end of life. When completed, the document states the types of care you would and would not want in the most commonly-occurring end-of-life care scenarios. In my experience, when patients and their family members are presented with the choices in a living will, they find them confusing and are often unsure how their choices will affect their lives. To help you through this confusion, I will briefly describe each of the choices most commonly included in a living will and some of the implications of those choices.

To be or not to be resuscitated. You may have seen a resuscitation on your favorite medical television show. It's the scene where the patient's monitor shows a flat line and begins to beep, signaling the patient has "passed away." Soon thereafter, the entire medical team rushes into the room and begins performing CPR and shocking the patient with the paddles. Do you want to be resuscitated with electric shock if you "pass away" while you are in the hospital? Or would you prefer to be what is known as a "do not resuscitate" (DNR), which means "do not attempt to revive me, let me pass away quietly." When making the resusitation decision, you will want to consider some of what we know about resusitation.

Occasionally resuscitations are successful and the patient goes on to have a normal life like those seen on TV. This is not as common as you might think. Statistically, patients who are resuscitated in the hospital under the best circumstances have a 22 percent chance of survival. Those who do survive are likely to suffer permanent brain damage caused by a lack of oxygen during the resusitation process. Resusitated patients are then placed on a ventilator. Without a living will that states under what circumstances you would like to discontinue life support, you could linger on the ventilator for years, and your family could be bankrupt by the cost of your care.

When making the resuscitation decision, you will also want to consider your age and current health status. Generally speaking, a resusitation performed on a 40-year-old who has a sudden heart attack (and is otherwise healthy) will be more successful than a resuscitation performed on someone who is very old or very ill. The resuscitation of an 85-year-old woman with a terminal illness could also cause her a great deal of pain and prolong her suffering. It is not uncommon during the resusitation process for patients to suffer lacerated organs, broken bones and burns. It is therefore important when making this decision that you take into consideration the status of your overall health, your prognosis, and the pain and suffering that are sure to come in the aftermath of this procedure.

Living on a respirator. Do you want to live on a respirator (a machine that breathes for you)? Do you want to live on a respirator indefinitely or only until it is clear that there is no hope of you breathing without the help of a machine? If you decide you would like to live on a respirator, who in your family will look after you while you are in a long-term care facility and how will your decision to live on a respirator effect their life? Can your family bear the financial ramifications of having a loved one in a nursing home? Answer these questions, make your decisions, and document them in your living will.

Artificial nutrition. In the event you are unable to chew or swallow food on your own for a long period, you may be given the option of being fed through a feeding tube (a tube placed in your stomach, through which liquid food is poured). Long-term tube feedings have physical, financial, and legal implications.

The physical side effects of tube feedings are diarrhea, which will require the need for frequent stool cleanings and increase your chances of developing bedsores. Tube feedings can also produce high blood sugar and hospital-induced diabetes. If you are incapacitated and your life is sustained by a feeding tube, you may need to be placed in a long-term care facility, and your assets could be turned over to that facility. If you return home, you may require private nurses to care for you.

The legal issues surrounding tube feedings have made national news. Perhaps you have heard the stories of Karen Ann Quinlan or Terry Schiavo. In each of those cases, long and painful court battles were fought before family members were allowed to discontinue tube feedings. Family members were not allowed to stop the feedings because of family disagreements and state laws that prohibited stopping the feedings without intervention from the courts.

Some of the questions you will want to ask and answer in this area are "Do you want to be fed artificially should you become unable to eat and swallow on your own?" "Do you want to be fed and sustained indefinitely or only until it is clear you will never recover from your illness?" The decision to start artificial nutrition is probably best based on your prognosis and how you would like to spend the rest of your life.

Antibiotics. Antibiotics can prolong life for a short time if an infection is bringing the end nearer, faster. At the end of life, antibiotics are generally not considered curative; they are used to extend life for a few days. If you are very near the end and antibiotics would extend your life by several hours, do you want them?

When making all of these choices you will want to consider:

- How much pain and suffering the choice will cause and for how long

- The type of treatments you want if there is every chance you will recover

- The type of treatments you want if there is a small chance you will recover

- The type of treatments you want if there is no real chance you will recover

- The type of care you will require based on your choice

- What is the cost of that care.

- What life be would be like for you and your loved ones after you make the choice

- How you want to live your life

- How you don't want to live your life

Completing the Paperwork

To obtain copies of the medical power of attorney and living will documents you can visit your local hospital or hospice where a patient representative or social worker will have standardized forms that meet your state's requirements. Either of these professionals will be able explain some of the choices to you and outline your state's procedures for properly filing the documents. If, at that point, you still have questions you can ask to speak with the palliative care nurse (a nurse who has been extensively trained in end-of-life care issues) and have your questions answered by an expert.

You can also get copies of a medical power of attorney and living will online. Two of the easiest sites to use are www.doyourproxy.com (has free documents) and www.lawdepot.com. Of course, you can also consult your attorney; however, this is an expensive option for a very inexpensive process. An attorney is not needed to complete these forms. However, these forms are a part of your estate planning and you may want to inform your attorney that you have completed them. You will want to have copies placed in your file along with your other estate planning documents. After you have made your choices and the documents are signed and notarized, there are just a few more steps you need to take to complete this process:

Your role as team leader:

- Discuss your wishes with everyone you feel should be involved in this process.

- Create a card for your wallet that informs members of the healthcare team that you have a healthcare proxy and a living will and where these documents are located.

- If your wishes change, change your documents and let everyone know your wishes have changed.

- Give copies of the documents to your proxy, the person who would be called in the event of an emergency, and to your primary care physician.

- Talk over your wishes with your primary care provider and ensure she supports your choices. If she doesn't, find a doctor that will.

A Story About What Happens When Advanced Care Directives Are Not Followed

The most memorable case I can recall of a doctor not following the instructions set out in a living will is the case of Mary the ballerina. Mary must have been quite something when she was dancing; she had been asked by special invitation to dance for the Queen of England. At 80 years old and completely unable to care for herself she didn't have one wrinkle in her porcelain skin. She had jet-black, thick, wavy hair and surprisingly well-toned muscles. She really was an amazingly beautiful woman.

Mary's late husband had been very wealthy and he had a team of lawyers prepare all of their estate documents before he died. He wanted to ensure Mary would be well taken care of after his passing. Together, they completed a living will and appointed their son Michael, to be their healthcare proxy.

Mary's living will specifically expressed refusal of a feeding tube. She did not want her body violated with a feeding tube or any other device that would spoil her natural beauty.

When Mary could no longer swallow on her own, her doctor suggested a permanent feeding tube be placed. Of course, Michael refused the tube in accordance with his mother's wishes. The doctor was not at all happy about Michael's refusal. He could not accept that Mary herself had refused a tube even after being presented with the signed and notarized documents.

The doctor shared with me that he felt Michael was waiting for Mary to pass on so he could get her money. This was not at all the case; Mary and her husband had given Michael his inheritance after the birth of his third child when he and his wife believed they had completed their family. Michael, his wife, and each of their three children were given a very large sum of money to avoid a situation in which there might appear to be a conflict of interest by putting Michael or his family members in the will. Michael clearly had no financial stake in Marys passing. It was also clear he was devoted to her care. He visited his mother everyday while she was in the hospital and he had managed all of her home care needs for over ten years. However, the doctor didn't see it that way.

One evening after Michael went home, the doctor had Mary wheeled down to the endoscopy suite and he placed a feeding tube in her abdomen.

When Michael arrived at the hospital the next morning, he was devastated to see the puncture wound in Mary's abdomen and a yellow rubber tube flapping against her porcelain skin. It clearly spoiled her physical beauty, something Mary never wanted. The doctor violated Mary's wishes, her body, and the law. To perform a treatment on a person who does not want that treatment without a court order is legally battery, a chargeable offense.

Michael sprang into action to protect his beloved mother. After a court proceeding, the tube was removed and a restraining order was issued, preventing the doctor from ever treating Mary again. Mary experienced an unwanted procedure; her family experienced the stress and the financial consequences of hiring an attorney and attending a court proceeding at what was already a very difficult time in their lives. This was a nightmare for them. This should not have happened, but it did, and it does happen. I have seen things like this on more than one occasion. We all need a strong advocate and a living will to protect our wishes.

Professional Advocates/Case Managers

Case managers are nurses who have specialized training in organizing and facilitating the delivery of patient care. There has recently been an increased demand for the services of case managers because healthcare is complicated and patients are often confused and unsure of which decisions are best. In order to respond to their patients' need for help, insurers, employers and hospitals hire case managers to help patients make the best healthcare decisions and to gather information that could spare their patients unnecessary or wrong treatments. In doing so, employers, insurance companies and the hospitals save hundreds of thousands of dollars that would have been spent if the patients made a poor choice or were harmed be a medical error. Employers especially benefit when patients get through the healthcare system safely and can return to work in a timely fashion and they are not injured by a wrong treatment. Safe healthcare delivery saves everyone money. Some of the many functions performed by the case manager are to:

- Ensure communication between patients and providers

- Prevent overlap of services

- Facilitation of second opinions

- Help avert injuries that could come about because of lack of communication

- Ensure care is being delivered according to set guidelines

- Coordinate discharge planning for home care services

- Get insurance clearance for providers, procedures, or hospitals that are not in the patients' plan under special circumstances.

Case managers and case management services may also specialize in different types of care. Some case managers specialize in insurance coverage, while others concentrate on coordinating care. Care coordinators will speak directly to your doctors to ensure you are getting the most appropriate care, care that is delivered in the most effient manner.

Because of the increased demand for case management services, private case management companies have emerged to meet the need. If you choose to hire a private case management service, be aware that you will have to shop for the type of services you need and can afford because the services offered by case management services vary. No matter how you acquire the services of a professional case manager or the type of services they provide this group of professionals can be very powerful professional advocates and very helpful members of *YOUR* Healthcare Team.

Your role as team leader:

- Call your health insurance company and ask what case management services they offer subscribers and become familiar with those services.

- In the event you are admitted to the hospital, ask to speak to the hospital's case manager. If she coordinates care (that is, she talks to providers about your care plan to assure appropriateness of care), and she can help you to get the care and services you will need after discharge from the hospital, ask her to be a member of your team. Because of the importance of this role, many hospitals will automatically assign you a case manager. If this is the case, ask to speak to her and discuss her role on your team. Ask how you can make the best use of her services.

- If you can afford private case management services and you need help coordinating your care (that is not forthcoming from your insurance company) seek the services of a private case manager.

- There are many different types of services available. Shop around for the company that will provide the help you need to care for yourself or your loved ones.

CHAPTER SEVEN

Your Personal Healthcare Record: (PHR) An Important Member Of *YOUR* Healthcare Team

"Nobody can do it for you."
Ralph Cordiner

No doubt you have seen your doctors writing in your healthcare record when you go in for a visit. Every healthcare provider you see creates a record of your care in a "chart." In the chart, the provider documents your complaints, your vital signs, test results and his or her treatment recommendations.

In addition to recording your current complaints and medical history, your medical record has clerical and administrative functions. The information contained in your medical record is translated into code numbers and given to your insurance company. The carrier then reviews your records to determine if the care you received was "customary and/or necessary." Your carrier then goes on to make billing, payment, and treatment decisions based upon what is written in your chart.

The medical record is also a central tool used in investigating medical legal injury claims. In a court of law, your medical record will be used to reveal how your injuries occurred; who may be responsible for causing your injuries; and if you will be compensated for your injuries. Clearly, your medical record is a very important member of *YOUR* Healthcare Team.

If you have seen more than one provider, you have more than one medical record. All of your records contain different pieces of your medical history; none of your records or your providers has a complete picture of your care. When more than one provider orders treatments without anyone monitoring the "big picture," multiple problems can and do occur. These problems include, but are not limited too, duplication of imaging and laboratory studies; dangerous medication combinations; and delays in care while records are transferred from one doctor to another.

Benefits of Having a Personal Healthcare Record

A personal healthcare record (PHR) is a is a complete record of your care that you assemble and keep in your possession. You do so by collecting your records and test results from all of your providers and storing them in one location. When you have a PHR, you can avoid many problems inherent to our current method of record keeping. Some of the other benefits of maintaining a PHR are:

- You have constant and free access to your healthcare information (many healthcare providers charge a fee to duplicate your records).

- Medical records can be lost in natural disasters or when doctors close their practices. By maintaining a PHR you can ensure the safety of your records.

- You help prevent treatment delays that occur while waiting for records to be gathered.

- You can help to prevent duplication of services.

- You can share information with providers about the care you have received by referring to your own documented history.

- You will be knowledgeable, well organized, proactive, and accurate.

- You will foster feelings of respect from members of **YOUR** Healthcare Team.

- You can refer to providers' instructions for prescriptions, tests, and treatments.

- You can track appointments, vaccinations, and other wellness services.

- You can record your progress toward specific health-related goals over time and review your progress.

- You can review insurance claims and will have the information you need to discuss your case with insurance providers if necessary.

- You will receive safer, more efficiently delivered care.

Forty percent of Americans indicate they have some sort of PHR, whether it is a filed in a drawer or stored on a computer disk. It is becoming increasingly popular for patients to contract with electronic medical record services so that their records can be retained and accessed online. Whatever format you decide to keep your medical records in your PHR should to include:

- Personal identification, including name and birth date

- Emergency contacts

- Allergies or any sensitivities

- Health insurance information

- Current medications and doses

- Your medical conditions

- Immunizations

- Recent exams and testing reports

- Names, addresses, and phone numbers of all of your providers including their specialties

- Surgeries

- Important events (for example, frequency of dialysis or regular blood transfusion) with scheduled dates and times

- Living will and healthcare proxy contact information.

- Family hereditary conditions

- Eye and dental records

- Organ donor authorization

- Correspondence between you and your providers

- Current educational materials (or appropriate Web links) relating to your health

- Anything else you feel is important to document

Steps to Creating and Maintaining Your PHR

Your role as team leader:

- Call all of your providers, including any specialists you have seen, and request copies of your records.

- If possible, obtain your pediatric records. They will contain your immunizations and a record of any childhood diseases and treatments.

- Contact the hospitals where you were a patient and ask for copies of your records.

- Give a copy of your PHR to your emergency contact and your advocate (if they are different people) in case of emergency. For privacy reasons, place these copies of your records in a sealed envelope to be opened only in case of emergency.

You do not have to gather all of your records at once. You can wait until the next time you visit the doctor and simply ask for a copy. Then, each time you access the healthcare system, get copies of your newly-created records.

Each provider and medical facility will have its own procedures and fees for copying medical records. The costs for records can only be for copying the records – not for the records themselves that is because in accordance with federal regulations your records belong to you and the provider. If you want your insurance company's records, you will need to contact your insurance company to request them.

Once you have your records, the simplest and possibly the easiest way to organize the information is to place everything in a three-ring binder that allows for chronological additions. You may want to divide the binder into one section for each member of your family and then organize each section by disease processes and dates. Or maybe you want each member of the family to have his or her own binder. It's your choice.

Electronic PHRs

If you decide to contract with an electronic medical records company, you will not need to have physical hard copies of your records because you will be able to access your records from any place with Internet service. You will be able to download your information to a computer or handheld device, your medical records will quite literally be at your fingertips.

You should be aware that thieves are now stealing medical identities. If the thiefs' provider alters your record, his care will be entered into your record and that could cause you a great deal of trouble. Say for example the thief has her appendix removed and this is documented in your medical record. Sometime thereafter you present to the emergency room with a ruptured appendix. If the doctors in the ER review your medical records and see a notation indicating you have already had your appendix removed will anyone think to check to see if you have an extra appendix? No, they will rule out the diagnosis and that could cost you your life. What if the thief has six months of physical therapy, she could exhaust your rehabilitation benefits for the year. The take home message here is, if you choose to maintain an electronic health record, you will want to choose a secure service and periodically monitor your online medical records for accuracy and to ensure no one else is receiving treatment at your expense.

Medical Record Errors

Your medical records are the primary source of communication between all the members of **YOUR** Healthcare Team. Your record tells team members what was and was not done in your case, and they suggest what should be done next. Doctors, nurses, nurse practitioners, therapists, insurance companies, case managers, and others read your records and rely on them for accurate information. If the information recorded in your chart is wrong, it can cause numerous problems, including doctors making a wrong diagnosis based upon reading wrong information in your chart. You could receive wrong tests and procedures or you could even be scheduled to have a wrong surgery based upon wrong information.

In an online doctors' forum I recently read, the doctors were discussing errors they found in their own charts. One doctor reported he had a degenerative nervous system disorder. His provider incorrectly charted that he had multiple brain tumors. The doctors' insurance company subsequently refused to pay for his degenerative nervous system treatments because his chart said he had multiple brain tumors. Another doctor reported that his doctor wrote in his chart that he had a stroke, although he never complained of symptoms even vaguely related to a stroke. Yet another physician shared a story of having to replace the entire medical record system in an office practice he bought because the old system was filled with errors and as such the system could not be relied upon to provide accurate information. Clearly, if physicians are at risk encountering errors in their record keeping systems we are all at risk of encountering an error in our own medical records

There are many types of medical record errors and they happen everyday. Personally, I cannot remember the last time I read a medical record that did not contain at least one error. In this section, I discuss several types of medical record errors and how you can protect yourself from them.

Filing errors. This type of error involves entering orders and test results in the wrong person's chart. In this example you have been admitted to the hospital and your doctor is treating both you and your roommate. The doctor intends to order lab tests for your roommate; however, he pulls the wrong chart from the chart rack because they both have the same room number printed on them, and they are placed next to each other in the chart rack. As a result, he accidentally enters your roommate's orders into your chart. The lab will now be drawing blood from you that was supposed to be taken from your roommate. Your roommate's tests and care based on those tests will be delayed.

Things could have been much worse, the doctor could have entered orders for an invasive procedure or surgery, and you could have received either prep work or the procedure itself because of a filing error. Filing errors are easy errors to make, and they happen all the time in paper charting systems. The question then becomes what can you do to protect yourself from an error in your medical record?

Your role as team leader:
- While in the hospital you or your advocate should ask your doctor what your treatment plan is for the day and record that information on the "Provider Visit Flow Sheet" provided at the end of this chapter.

- If anyone attempts to perform any test or procedure that was not discussed with you or your advocate, await clarification before consenting to the procedure.

Lack of truthfulness. Some providers do not tell the truth. I'm sorry to say it, but it's true. Providers document visits that they never made so they can be paid for the visit or to avoid having others know they did not actually see the patient. Providers also add or subtract information after problems have occurred to protect themselves from a potential malpractice suit. A dishonest report will influence the decisions others make when they assume what they are reading is true. Accurate and truthful charting is very important to your safety.

Your role as team leader:

- In the outpatient setting, ask your provider if she would read out loud the notes she entered into your chart during the visit. If the doctor does not have time to do so, ask to have the office nurse read the chart to you after each visit and get copies of your records.

- When in the hospital, ask to read your chart on a regular basis.

If you find an error in your chart, bring it to the attention of the provider who made the error and have the provider correct it. If they refuse, you will want to talk with hospital administration and press the issue. Remember: your safety and possibly reimbursement for your care depend in part on the information in your chart.

Poor handwriting. We have all wondered how anyone could read a doctors' handwriting. Poor handwriting is a very serious and a very common problem. If something in the chart is misunderstood, the potential problems are innumerable: wrong medications, wrong doses, delayed or wrong treatments, billing errors, and payment denials, to name just a few.

Your role as team leader:

- While in the hospital, you or your advocate should write down what your providers say to you on the "Provider Visit Flow Sheet."

- Periodically ask to review your chart and compare your recollection of the events against what is recorded in your medical record.

If you cannot understand the medical language or if the handwriting is poor, do not be embarrassed to ask to have the patient representative (or another designated professional) review the chart with you and to help you understand what is written.

Your medical record is a very important member of **YOUR** Healthcare Team and it is important that the information it contains is accurate. This may require some work from you; however, it is well worth the effort to protect your health and safety.

Provider Visit Flow Sheet

Date and Time of Visit	Name of Provider	Comments About Exam	Test Results	Next Steps (Labs, tests, therapy...)

Keep this flow sheet at your bedside while in the hospital for easy access. Use it to help you keep up with each provider's comings and goings, along with what he said and did. If you need more copies of the sheet feel free to make copies and be sure to make this document a part of your PHR.

CHAPTER EIGHT

Beware of Diagnostic Errors

"Our profession, after all, deals partly with guesswork."

Paul Beeson, M.D.

Up to 40 Percent of Medical Diagnosis are Wrong!

A diagnostic error occurs when the patient is given a wrong diagnosis. Missed and wrong diagnosis are among the most common types of medical mistakes. The evaluation of 53 autopsy studies found up to 40 percent of the cases reviewed had a major diagnostic error. The rates of diagnostic error are even higher in emergency rooms and in intensive care units, where decisions must be made very quickly. In a 1997 study conducted by the National Patient Safety Foundation, again, up to 40 percent of the patients surveyed stated they or someone they knew had been involved in an incident involving a diagnostic error.

Both patients and providers contribute to the making of a wrong diagnosis. In this chapter I will discuss some of those reasons and the types of diagnostic errors, which include but at not limited too:

Types of Diagnostic Errors

A wrong diagnosis. The diagnosis you are given is inaccurate and has on relationship to the condition you actually have.

You are not sick. You are diagnosed with an illness when you do not have an illness.

Missed diagnosis. You are told you do not have a illness when, in fact, you do have an illness. The doctor "missed" the diagnosis.

Missed underlying disease. In this scenario the provider fails to diagnosis the underlying cause of your chief complaint. If, for an example, you are given the diagnosis of headache and the doctor fails to diagnose the high blood pressure that is causing the headache, the high blood pressure becomes a missed underlying disease.

Missed complications. Many diseases have complications; for example, complications of diabetes include ocular disease, kidney failure, and cardiovascular disease. If the doctor does not screen the patient for these complications and they are allowed to progress without intervention the patient will eventually develop the complications associated with their primary diagnosis because in part, the doctor failed to properly screen for and detect these underlying problems.

Missed medication side effects. Both prescription and over-the-counter medications have side effects. For example, an over dose of non-aspirin pain relievers can cause liver failure. Use of steroids can cause brittle bones and mental agitation. The list of medication side effects goes on and on. Medication side effects can be overlooked and diagnosed as a new disorder, when, in fact, the symptoms could be relieved by stopping or changing the medication.

A Story About Medication Side Effects and a Missed Diagnosis

One of my nursing students, who I will call Holly, recently came to me in tears. Her 17- year-old daughter had developed glaucoma, which was getting worse. Holly had taken her daughter to three ophthalmologists, and not one of them could find a reason for her daughters' problem. It seemed that without divine intervention blindness was all but certain. As I listened to her story I remembered her daughter had a history of really bad allergies. I asked, "Has your daughter been taking allergy medications?" She replied, "Yes, she has been on antihistamines for years." I reminded Holly that antihistamines are a group of drugs known to contribute to the development of glaucoma. Holly became angry, frustrated, and confused all at once. She said, "That can't be, why would they give my daughter a drug that would cause glaucoma?"

I explained, "They did not give her a drug that would cause glaucoma, they gave her a drug to treat her allergies. One of the potential side effects of that group of drugs is glaucoma." My point was that no one meant to hurt her daughter, but that all medications have the potential to harm you, that's just the way it is. Each of us needs to know this and be on the look out for the side effects of our medications.

I spoke with Holly recently, she called to thank me again for helping with her with her daughters' case. They stopped the antihistamines, and her daughters' vision was very much improved. Yeah!! A happy ending.

There are many reasons why doctors choose the wrong diagnosis and there are things patients say and do that contribute to a wrong diagnosis. Below I have outlined some of these things and given you the steps you can take to increase the probability you'll get a correct diagnosis. Let's get started.

Provider Reasons for Making a Wrong Diagnosis

Lack of time. The average length of an office visit is 15 minutes. This means the doctor has to process a good deal of information in a very short period of time, making it easy to overlook or to forget things. The short office visit leaves no time to research and learn more about the patient's complaints. In short, rapid-fire visits increase the probability of getting a wrong diagnosis.

Two diseases have similar symptoms. If the provider has to choose between two conditions with similar symptoms, she could choose the wrong one .

There may be two diseases going on at once. If you have two disorders, one may be overlooked and go undiagnosed and untreated.

Inability to understand the patient. When the doctor does not understand the patient for any reason, the information the patient gives can be misunderstood. The patient could easily be given a wrong diagnosis.

The doctor did not know about the disorder. There are more than 20,000 human diseases. Doctors will know the most common diseases and the ones they see most often. They will not know about disorders they have never seen or been taught about. Because the doctor cannot know everything, unusual and unfamiliar disorders are sometimes missed.

Provider skill level. Some doctors have highly developed diagnostic skills; they are knowledgable; they have experience;

and they trust their instincts. Others are not so well endowed, and thus they are not as skillful in the art of making an accurate diagnosis. In addition, doctors who are experts in their area of specialty will be better at diagnosing disorders in their area of expertise than someone who is not an expert in diagnosing the disorder.

Over-publicized diseases. Diseases that receive a lot of attention and/or publicity tend to be over-diagnosed in the doctor's office.

Doctor bias. When providers routinely see a disease in their practice, they may habitually assign that diagnosis to patients without looking any further for an alternative cause of the patients complaints. The doctor may overlook additional symptoms that would lead to a different diagnosis.

Rare or unusual diagnosis. When a condition is rare or unusual for the age and sex of the patient, the diagnosis may be overlooked or missed all together. Many women, for example, are misdiagnosed when they present to the emergency room with a heart attack because of the persistant myth that says heart attacks are rare in women. Furthermore, women tend to present with unusal symptoms when they experience a myocardial infarction; as a result, the diagnosis is missed.

The diagnosis does not have a definitive diagnostic test. Without tests to confirm or refute a diagnosis there may be no way to be certain the diagnosis is correct.

Cost. Some doctors will avoid expensive tests and tests that are not covered by your insurance company in order to reduce costs. In addition, the doctor may not order tests that diagnose rare conditions because he may believe there is a very low probability of you having the disorder. This works well for the large majority of patients, but fails for the small percentage of patients who have rare conditions. This minority could have their ailment diagnosed had cost not prohibit testing.

Mental illness. Patients who are mentally ill or confused and those who suffer with dementia are difficult to diagnose because they are unable to clearly communicate their symptoms. As always, communication is an essential element in every area of healthcare safety.

Things Patients Do that Can Lead to a Wrong Diagnosis

Patients Withhold information. Patients withhold information because they are uncomfortable discussing "personal problems" and because they are afraid of the consequences of telling the truth. Not revealing information related your condition could result in a wrong diagnosis and delay proper treatment.

In the following example, a man goes to the doctor with palpations and chest pain and his doctor cannot determine the cause of his problem. The doctor orders more tests and procedures and requests a second opinion. All the while, the patient has a secret: he is addicted to cocaine. Cocaine causes palpations and its abuse can lead to a heart attack, stroke, seizures, and death. Because the doctor does not know about the cocaine, he cannot properly diagnosis and treat the patient or help him get into a recovery program that may save his life. Withholding information can lead to a wrong diagnosis, delay proper treatment and could have lethal consequences!! There is a saying that goes "You are only as sick as your secrets." It fits here.

Your role as team leader:

- Choose a doctor you can trust, one with whom you can be honest.

- Tell your doctor about any activities or symptoms you have that you believe are related to your medical condition.

- Volunteer the information even if you feel the information is personal and should be kept private. Even if no one asks, if you feel the information you are withholding bears on your medical condition, tell your doctor. This will help you to get an accurate diagnosis and timely treatment.

Sometimes patients delay reporting symptoms. Patients wait weeks, months, and even years to report symptoms, because they do not want to go to the doctor or because they are afraid of receiving a diagnosis and treatment plan.

Your role as team leader:

- If something goes on without improvement seek help.

- Keep a record of and report your symptoms using the O.L.D.C.A.R.T.S format. This will help you to give a complete and coherent account of symptoms you may have had for a long time

- Research your symptoms on a symptom checker and report your findings to the doctor.

Sometimes patients are hypochondriacs. Dr. Paul Tornier once said, "Many ordinary illnesses are nothing but the expression of a serious dissatisfaction with life." Sometimes patients have multiple and frequent complaints and their doctors are unable to diagnose a physical condition. In some of these cases, the patients are thought to be hypochondriacs. When a patient is labeled a hypochondriac, high suspicion among healthcare providers erupts that there are emotional or psychological problems that are generating physical discomfort. This is not at all uncommon. Something as simple as a headache can be the result of constant worry. To some degree, all of our physical complaints have a psychological effect on our lives.

There are, however, potentially very serious problems associated with frequent trips to the doctor's office. Among them is that sooner or later the patient will be given a diagnosis, possibly for a condition that does not exist. Patients who frequent the doctor's office have the likilhood of being exposed to tests and procedures that have their own risk factors.

Your role as team leader:

- If you find yourself frequently at the doctor's office for one complaint or another and there is no clear diagnosis, consider seeing a therapist to be evaluated for stress, anxiety, depression, and loneliness. All of these are common causes of physical discomfort and require their own treatment plan to bring relief.

Sometimes patients try to commit fraud to get time off work and to gain other benefits. Faking is dangerous and exposes the faker to the possibility of medical error. In this example, the patient consents to and has an unnecessary CAT scan because the doctor is trying to find a reason for his abdominal pain (which he doesn't have). Sounds harmless right? Well let's see about that. The dye or contrast used during the test sends the patient into kidney failure. That's right – contrast dye can damage the kidney, possibly for life. Patients have also been known to have fatal allergic reactions to contrast agents. All medications, tests, treatments, and procedures can harm as well as help. The medical system is not to be entered into lightly. Be careful and do not expose yourself risk.

Your role as team leader:
- Do not fake symptoms for any reason.

- Do not expose yourself to unnecessary test and procedures.

Sometimes patients push providers for unneeded medications. While this is not a wrong diagnosis, insisting the doctor give you a prescription that is not necessary leads to the wrong treatment and exposes you to possible medication side effects that can alter your life. Over using antibiotics can cause resistance to them, and they may be rendered ineffective when you really do need them. Over using antibiotics also leads to the development of a very serious infectious gastric disease known as C-Difficile. And, last but not least, contiued overuse of antibiotics will decrease the functioning of your immune system. If your provider feels you do not need an antibiotic, it is best to accept his opinion and try other measures to treat your condition.

Likewise, the over use of pain medication can cause life-long issues with addiction and make existing problems like depression and bowel disorders much worse. If your doctor does not want to give you a medication and has a sound rationale – a reason you can understand that synchs with your honest feelings about what is going on – you will be safer if you listen to the provider.

Your role as team leader:

- Take antibiotics only when really needed.

- If you find yourself seeking mood-altering substances in the doctor's office you may want to get help. Addiction is a horrible condition that keeps you chained to a doctor or an illegal supplier.

- If you need help dealing with an addiction, get it. Set yourself free from the prescription pad.

Laboratory Errors and Misdiagnosis

Doctors rely upon laboratory tests to confirm or deny a diagnosis and to develop proper treatment plans. It is of vital importance that you have accurate test results if you are going to be accurately diagnosed and receive appropriate care.

Laboratory error has been estimated to occur in 1 to 3 percent of all laboratory test results. A 1 percent error rate in a laboratory that reports 1,000,000 tests per year equals 10,000 errors per year; 830 errors per month; 30 errors per day, and 1.25 errors per hour! A Johns Hopkins Hospital study of 6,171 slides found a 1.4 percent error rate in examining cells referred for cancer diagnosis. Of the 86 misdiagnosed patients in the study, 20 had non-cancerous tumors, which were diagnosed as cancerous. These patients probably received treatment for cancers they did not have. In this section, I discuss types of laboratory errors, why they occur, and the questions you can ask to help prevent a laboratory error from happening in your case.

Types of Laboratory Errors

Inaccurate results. Sometimes the machines in the lab simply gets it wrong and they produce an inaccurate result.

Test contamination. Specimens are considered to be contaminated when they are mixed with things with which they should not be mixed and when they are improperly stored. If a specimen should be refrigerated and it is not, the specimen can be contaminated or spoiled and will yield an incorrect result.

Mislabeling of sample. The wrong person's name was placed on the specimen and thus two people have their results confused.

False positives and false negatives. An example of this sort of error is receiving a positive pregnancy test when you are not pregnant; this is considered a false positive. In a false negative, the patient is told she is not pregnant when she really is pregnant. Most laboratory tests have conditions under which they will give a false positive or a false negative result.

Misinterpretation. Tissue samples are looked at under a microscope by a pathologist or technician, if the person looking at the sample misinterprets what he or she sees you will receive a misdiagnosis or a missed diagnosis.

Needless Laboratory Tests. While not actually a medical error, needless tests can lead to other errors. A false positive may lead to more tests and procedures and expose the patient to the potential side effects of those tests and procedures. A false positive of an unnecessary test could lead to the treatment of a condition the patient does not have.

A study that reviewed 4,600 diagnostic tests found one-third of the patients in the study had submitted to tests that were not recommended, and were even advised against under professional guidelines. Urinalysis, electrocardiograms, and x-rays were inappropriately ordered for up to 46 percent of the patients. Needless testing increases our national healthcare costs by as much as $194 million a year.

Your role as team leader:
- Ask the following questions whenever lab tests are ordered for you:

Questions to Ask When Laboratory Tests are Ordered

- **What is the test for and why do we need these results?**

You will want to ask if the test is needed to diagnose, monitor, or treat your condition. You will also want to know if the test results will change your diagnosis or treatment plan. Generally speaking, if a test does not contribute to your diagnosis or treatment plan, it is an unnecessary test. Asking this questions could help prevent unnecessary testing, unnecessary treatments, pain, additional costs, and the stress of waiting for test results.

- **What will the results tell us?**

Ask your provider to explain to you in terms you can understand what the test will tell *YOUR* Healthcare Team;

too much iron, too little hemoglobin, too much salt, too little water, and so on. Ask how the results will influence your care. Again, if the test does not serve a useful purpose or give you useful information, you may want to forgo it.

- **How do I prepare for the test?**

Ask the doctor or the nurse how to prepare for the test. Ask if you will need to fast or stop any of your medications before the test. You will also want to know if there are any special times or ways in which you should collect or store specimens at home. Many tests and procedures have preprinted literature to guide patients though the preparation process in a step-by-step manner. Ask the nurse for a copy of any educational materials that accompany the test. Improper test preparation yields inaccurate test results and can lead to a wrong treatment plan. Improper preparation could also create a need to repeat the test and the hassle of having the test re-approved by the insurance company, taking time off work, and exposure to more risk.

- **Who will perform the test?**

Tissue sampling may require the expertise of a surgeon. If the tissue is improperly collected, you could be injured during the collection; the procedure could be more painful than it needs to be; and the sample collected could be insufficient or otherwise unacceptable. To prevent or limit these types of errors, you will want to choose a provider who has a good deal of experience and a proven track record of safe practice.

- **Is the test painful?**

When patients are afraid and anxious, it can be difficult to perform procedures and their anxiety increases their risk of injury during the procedure. It is safer to perform a procedure when the patient is relaxed and able to cooperate with those performing the test. If you think you will need help relaxing or you will need something for pain, ask for it. If it is not customary to give pain medication, but you know you are not the best with handling pain, ask for special consideration in your case.

- **Should the test be performed by a specialty lab?**

For routine testing, most labs will be fine; however, some tests require special technology or training to properly perform the test. If you are having a test that your doctor refers to as unusual or "special testing," she may refer you to a specialty lab. Sometimes doctors will not know whether or not a test should be performed at a specialty lab. For an extra measure of safety, call the laboratory where you plan to have the test performed and ask the technicians if the test is routinely performed at their lab. If not, contact your insurance company to locate the lab with which they have contracted to perform the test.

- **How often will the test need to be performed?**

Some tests are a part of the treatment plan. For example if you are taking a mediation that has "pril" ending you should have your kidney function monitored at regular intervals; there are many common medications that require regular laboratory testing in order to ensure your safety while taking them. You will also want to keep track of your test results and compare your current results to your previous results each time the test is done. When test results vary widely without a clear cause, you should suspect a laboratory error.

- **Can we recheck the results to make sure they are accurate?**

When current lab results differ vastly from previous results and when your test results do not match your physical symptoms, there may be a laboratory error. In this example, the lab report says Mr. Jones is anemic. The symptoms of anemia include weakness, fatigue and paleness. Mr. Jones, on the other hand, is strong, has plenty of energy, works out everyday, and has great color. In this case, he is probably not anemic and should have the blood test repeated.

- **When will we get the results?**

An overlooked lab result could cause a delay in treatment and allow a treatable disorder to progress into something worse. To prevent this from happening, call your provider and request your test results if you are not notified of the results when you were told you would be. In today's busy world, things do get missed, and you do not want this to happen to you.

- **What steps will we take after we get the test results?**

What comes next? Will you need blood transfusions? Will future testing be based on the results of these tests? Knowing the answers to these questions will help you plan for the future. Having these answers will allow you time to research the next steps in the process.

A Story About Laboratory Error

Recently my daughter called me from her doctor's office to tell me the doctor said she "didn't have any white blood cells." I silently panicked thinking, "Oh goodness, my baby has cancer!!" I immediately began inwardly and silently screaming. What I said outwardly was, "Wasn't your last blood test normal?" She answered "yes." I told her to have the nurse practitioner repeat the test. To reassure her, I reminded her she didn't have any of the symptoms that accompany that lab result and that all of her other lab tests were normal. She said her nurse practitioner had already suggested the test be repeated because she too thought there must be a lab error based on the previous results and her overall health status. The test was repeated and she is fine. Whew!!! What a relief.

CHAPTER NINE

Prepare for the Office Visit and Prevent a Diagnostic Error

"Prepare and prevent, don't repair and repent"
Author Unkown

You have Eighteen Seconds to Talk

The average length of an office visit with a primary care provider is fifteen minutes. Once the office visit begins, you have 18 seconds to talk before the doctor will interrupt you and begin asking questions. When a doctors starts asking questions that generally means he has made a tentative diagnosis. The questions he asks are to confirm or to rule out, (refute) his suspicions. So, in effect, you have 18 seconds to talk before the doctor makes a diagnosis upon which he is likely to act upon. This type of high-speed interview sets the stage for a missed or wrong diagnosis, inappropriate testing to confirm the wrong diagnosis, wrong medications, and more. Additionally, rapid-fire visits leave little time for patient education or development of treatment plans patients can understand, and will be willing to follow. To prevent the pitfalls of a wrong diagnosis, there needs to be clear, concise and accurate, communication between patients and their providers. This type of communication requires preparation. Using the lessons you have already learned in this book, you will so see you already have all of the tools you need to help your provider make the right diagnosis.

Your role as team leader:

- **Monitor your symptoms and associated factors**. Record your findings on the O.L.D.C.A.R.T.S worksheet in the Appendix of this book.

- **Practice "telling your story" before the office visit.** Practicing will help you to tell your story in a concise and all-inclusive manner and in a way that will take only seconds for you to articulate. This will leave time for questions and answers, further exploring symptoms, education, and developing care plans.

- **Bring your assessments with you to your visits**. Having your symptoms documented on the O.L.D.C.A.R.T.S worksheet in a language the doctor understands and respects will help her to review your complaints in a systematic fashion and give her the opportunity to review your complaints in writing. Writing your symptoms down will also help you remember everything you want to say and to ensure nothing is overlooked.

- **Tell the doctor what you think**. Several research studies found that patients were more accurate than their doctors when diagnosing themselves with common ailments. Be sure to tell your doctor what you think is wrong with you. In most cases you will be right.

- **Volunteer information; do not wait to be asked.** Your doctor may not remember to ask you about symptoms that are important to making the proper diagnosis, or you may offer a symptom that completely changes his or her idea of what is going on in your case. Volunteer information, especially if you think something is connected to your problem, even if he or she doesn't ask you about it. Share information even if it makes you feel embarrassed or uncomfortable. Doctors are people too; they understand the human condition and have probably heard the same thing you are going to tell them at least once. And, if they haven't, here is their opportunity to learn and grow by hearing something new.

- **Check your symptoms on a symptom checker before you go to the doctor's office.** Bring a list of possible diagnosis from the symptom checker located on a credible site. By now you know my favorites:

www.About.com

www.Mayoclinic.com

www.WebMD.com

www.symptomchecker.com

- **Review the possibilities associated with your symptoms (possible diagnosis) before going to the doctor's office.** When you are familiar with the possibilities, you can help the doctor chose the diagnosis that most closely matches your case. (Read more about symptom checkers in Chapter Two).

- **Bring your personal healthcare record.** If you are visiting a new provider, you will want to bring your records with you for the doctor to review and you will want to have your past medical history made part of the new providers' files. Knowing your history and the results of previous testing saves time and money and prevents delays that could occur while waiting for your records to be assembled and delivered to the new doctor's office.

- **Bring any medicines you are taking or have stopped taking.** Once a year you and all of your providers should review all the medications you are taking. This will help determine if your medications or their side effects are related to your current symptoms and to ensure you are taking a safe combination of drugs. This process also gives each of your providers a list of your medications and their effectiveness, a list they should have before prescribing any new medications.

- **Bring your advocate.** Your advocate is an important source of support and an extra set of ears. You may need an extra set of ears because when we are under stress, (like the stress that occurs when the doctor gives us a new medical diagnosis of any kind) we often miss what is said to us after the "bad" news is delivered. You advocate can help you listen to and understand what transpired during the office visit. It's especially beneficial to bring your advocate to visits with a specialist and visits where you will be getting a second opinion. You'll also want your advocate to be present at appointments with surgeons in which you will discuss upcoming surgery and treatments needed after surgery that your advocate may be responsible to provide. When your advocate is present during the office visits she will later be able to help you review what was said and suggested during the visit and she'll be there to help you cope with the stress. Make every effort to schedule appointments for times when your advocate is available to go with you to the doctors office.

Once you are given a diagnosis, you may need help understanding what the diagnosis is and how it will affect your life. The answers to the following questions will help you understand your diagnosis, treatments, your treatment options, the risks and benefits of each option, and any lifestyles changes that may be required. Read the questions and decide which ones you need to ask in your situation. Some diagnosis have simple treatment options and will only require answers to a few of these questions. Other conditions are more involved and you will need the answers to many, if not all, of these questions before you can fully understand the ramifications of your new diagnosis. No matter which scenario presents itself, ask the questions you need answered and leave the rest. Like all of the other question sets in the book, these too, are available in the Appendix with space for you to fill in the provider's answers.

Questions To Help You Understand Your Diagnosis and Treatment Options

- **What is my diagnosis?**

- **What does it mean in plain English?**

- **Is additional testing needed before you are sure of the diagnosis or are you sure now?**

- **What are my treatment options?**

- **What are the benefits of each treatment option?**

- **Which option do you recommend considering my unique circumstances, my age, gender, culture, and my ability to tolerate the treatment?**

Always ask about the options. Doctors will usually suggest options with which they are familiar or the ones they prefer. Rarely is the doctor's preference the only option and it may not be the best choice for you. Explore your options by talking with the doctor about all of the choices and by doing your own research.

If you find discrpencies between the information your doctor gives you and other available options, ask your doctor why he prefers the option he suggested. Then, make a choice based on the most complete information available and what best suits your medical and personal needs.

- **What are the risks associated with my treatment options?**

- **In what percentage of cases is each of my options successful?**

- **What do you consider successful?**

- **Have you treated patients in the way you are suggesting?**

- **How are those patients doing now?**

If your doctor has suggested surgery or a major invasive procedure, you may want to speak to one or two of the doctors' other patients who had the same treatment and ask them how they are doing now. You may want to ask how the procedure has affected their lives.

- **How long does it take to get results from each of the treatment options?**

- **How many treatments will I need?**

- **Does my insurance cover the treatment you suggest?**

If the provider suggests a treatment that is not covered by your insurance and she considers it the best option (and you agree), call the case manager at the insurance company to ask that the treatment be approved. The case manager may have the ability to work out special terms and conditions under which you can have the treatment you need. Having the provider's office call and state the reasons why you need the treatment can be helpful in persuading the insurance company to consider paying for your treatment.

- **What are the treatment's side effects?**

- **How will we manage the side effects?**

- **Will I have pain and if so, how will we manage it?**

- **Is there a chance that someone else in my family will get or develop the same condition?**

Am I contagious? Is my condition genetic? If so, what should those affected do?

- **Should I see a specialist?**

- **Do you recommend anyone?**

- **How will this affect my life?**

- **What happens if I choose to have no treatment at all?**

Will I need; nursing care, family support, or physical therapy, help education or counseling?

- **Is there anything I should do to monitor myself?**

Should I take my blood pressure, monitor my blood sugar, check my weight, count my calories, or have routine laboratory work?

- **Is there anyone who can teach me to do those things?**

- **In your opinion, what is my prognosis? What is likely to happen to me in the course of this disease?**

- **Will I be able to work?**

- **How long will I be out of work?**

- **Can you help me complete my disability forms?**

- **Are there any natural therapies you would recommend to help me or that could alleviate the side effects of the treatments?**

Do you recommend massage, aromatherapy, vitamins, supplements, yoga, acupuncture, meditation, or a change in diet? How will they help me?

- **Are there any educational or support groups to help me through this?**

Good Follow-Up Care Could Mean Good Care

After you have made a treatment choice that you and your doctor can agree upon, it is important to follow the plan. When laboratory, diagositic tests, and other procredures are not completed properly it may be impossible for your doctor to properly treat your condition or to monitor your progress.

Your role as team leader:
Summarize and clarify. At the end of your appointment, be sure you understand your diagnosis, your treatment plan, medication changes, diet, and follow-up activities. The best way to do this is to repeat to your doctor your care instructions and clarify any misunderstanding before you leave the office.

If necessary, say "I don't understand." If you do not understand what was said say "I don't understand." Ask questions until you get answers you can understand.

If you think the doctor is wrong. If you do not believe the diagnosis you are given is correct, be honest. Tell the doctor "I really don't think we have the right diagnosis" and begin having a conversation about what to do next. Follow your instincts and get a second opinion. See Chapter Ten, "You May Need A Second Opinion" later in this book.

Ask for educational materials to take home with you. Your provider may have brochures or information packets or be able to refer you to websites and support groups. Read the materials and visit the sites or groups to learn more about how to manage your condition.

After you leave the office. If you do not understand the plan, chances are you will not follow it correctly or completely. If the plan is not followed correctly, tests and procedures may have to be rescheduled; you may lose time from work to repeat tests; and you may have to gain insurance approval for the procedure to be repeated. Improper follow-up can be very problematic. If you have *any* questions at all about your treatment plan, call the doctor's office or the facility performing your tests and ask the questions for which you need answers to ensure you get the plan right the first time.

If your symptoms get worse. If your symptoms get worse, call to find out if you will need to come back to the office; alter the treatment plan; stop the treatment; or start a new treatment. All of these options are possibilities if the plan is not working, or if you are getting worse. Call your provider and ask which option is best for you and your care.

If you cannot tolerate or just don't like your treatment plan. If you have unexpected or unmanageable side effects, call your provider or the pharamist to get instructions on what to do. Several options exist if you have difficulty tolerating medications. Some medications should be stopped slowly; some should be stopped right away; sometimes the dosage needs to be decreased. Call your doctor to find out which option is right for you. If you quit the treatment, let the doctor know so that he will not base future decisions on the belief that you completed the initial treatment If the provider thinks you're taking your medication and you're not, bad things can happen.

In this example, you go back to the doctor after being prescribed blood pressure medication and your blood pressure is still high. The doctor increases the medication dose, thinking the lower dose did not work (which it didn't because you didn't take it). Well…now you're afraid because your pressure is really high. You start taking the new medication at the higher dose and begin having severe side effects, so you stop taking the medication again. Soon thereafter, you end up in the ER with a stroke secondary to untreated blood pressure. You can totally avoid situations like this by being honest, communicating with your doctor, and developing a plan you will actually follow.

If you have another plan. Be honest about wanting to use or using natural or alternative therapies or some combination of what the doctor prescribed and natural therapies. Tell the provider you believe in natural therapies; that you are using them; and that you want to have them incorporated into your treatment plan.

This decision does not have to put you at odds with your doctor, even though doctors can be judgmental and standoffish toward patients who use natural therapies. Many doctors have been trained to be suspicious of natural therapies, and they are not given much, if any, training in this area. It is quite possible that you know more about your natural and cultural therapies than your doctor. That's okay, because you and the doctor can learn from one another.

In order to help ease any fears and apprehension your doctor may have, go to the office having researched your conditions and the therapies you are considering. Your doctor is more likely to work with you in a collaborative manner if he has printed information from respected sites about the therapies you are using.

Complete ordered tests. For various reasons patients do not complete ordered tests; lack of insurance coverage, time constraints, fear of the results, fear of the test itself, not having a ride after the procedure, and disbelief about the diagnosis are some of the reasons why patients do not complete suggested tests. If you told your doctor you would get the test done and later change your mind, discuss your reasons with the doctor and maintain an open line of communication between you and the doctor.

If you have tests done and do not hear from your doctor. Call for your test results. Don't assume no news is good news. Everyone is overworked and overwhelmed and things get missed. Don't forget to request a copy of your results for your PHR, and remember that now is the time to get a copy of your results without having to pay copying charges.

Take the inititive. If your treatment plan requires diet and exercise or any other type of lifestyle change, research your options and make choices. Choose which vegtables you will eat, which gym you will join, the type of exercise you will do, and so on.

If you can't afford the plan. Tell your doctor you can't afford the plan. If the doctor says you need a nurse at home, special equipment, or expensive medications that you cannot afford, you must admit you can't afford it. Then, ask what, if any, services are available to help you get the care you need. If you do not have insurance, call your state board of health and ask for a list of programs for state residents that are able to help you get the services you need.

If you cannot afford your medications. Call the drug companies that manufacture your medications and ask about their "compassionate use" program. These programs supply drugs at no or very low cost to consumers who cannot afford their medications. Also ask if you can take generic medications. Generic medications are non-name brand drugs that are less expensive than their name brand counter parts. Finally, Walgreens and Walmart (and perhaps others in your area) offer many common medications at very low prices.

If your doctor said you should see a specialist. Go see the specialist. Take your PHR, lab tests, x-rays, surgical reports, other materials related to your case with you.

Consider depression. This is really big news, so *please read the following section* if you are having trouble treating your current conditions or finding the right diagnosis. Please read on!!!

It may be depression: Up to 80 Percent of Patients are Depressed

According to a University of Colorado study, up to 80 percent of all office visits involve some degree of depression. Many people suffer the effects of depression without ever knowing they have it. Depression can masquerade as chronic fatigue, insomnia, agitation, stomach upsets, constipation, nausea, chest pain, headaches, constant pain, and more.

The World Health Organization reports that depression is the leading cause of disability among adults of all ages worldwide. It affects approximately 18.8 million Americans. Patients diagnosed with depression spend, on average, $4,246 per year on medical costs versus $2,371 spent by patients without depression. By 2020, it is projected that depression will be the number two cause of death in the country second only to heart disease.

Each of us is at risk of becoming depressed at one time or another for any number of reasons. The death of a loved one, loss of a job, prolonged separations, and financial problems can all bring about episodes of this crippling disease.

When depression is missed, left undiagnosed, and untreated it is reasonable to expect patients and their families will suffer needlessly. Depression is an awful disease for which there is treatment. Left unchecked, however, it can ruin lives and make many medical conditions worse than they need be.

Conditions That are Worsed by Depression

Heart diseases. Recent studies have shown one-fifth of all patients with heart disease suffer with depression. Depression can come after heart disease or it can be a contributory factor to the development of the disease. Canadian researchers found a significantly higher risk of death from cardiac disease one year after diagnosis in patients who were also depressed. This was true no matter what the level of heart disease – depression was more of a marker for death than the heart disease itself. Have you ever heard of someone dying from a broken heart? Of course you have. Untreated depression actually does kill.

High blood pressure: Depression increases your risk of developing high blood pressure. People who are depressed tend to smoke more, drink more, eat more, to be anxious, and they are ill-tempered and argumentative. When we eat poorly, smoke, drink, and have problems in our relationships we develop high blood pressure.

Diabetes: According to the American Diabetic Association, diabetics suffer from depression at rates three to four times higher than the general population. A 2004 Johns Hopkins study that tracked 11,615 patients without diabetes over six years found that "depressive symptoms" predicted the onset or development of Type II diabetes. The same study found that successfully treating diabetes may be tied to successfully treating depression. Depression causes overeating and cravings for sweet and fatty foods. Depression is also associated with feelings of fatigue and lethargy, which make it very difficult to exercise or even get out of bed. Overeating and little or no exercise are real barriers to successfully controlling diabetes.

Stroke, Parkinson's, and Alzheimer's disease: Up to 160,000 stroke patients annually experience a major depression. Depression rates range from 17-31 percent of patients with Alzheimer's disease and approximately 50 percent of patients with Parkinson's disease. Depression seriously affects the patient's ability to participate in their own recovery. Depressed patients eat too little or too much; sleep too little or too much; refuse to exercise; and have less hope and confidence in the future.

Exhaustion and fatigue: Depression is associated with feelings of exhaustion and fatigue, both of which make living life in general and healing from any medical condition more difficult. When we do not have the energy necessary to interact in relationships, we become isolated, suffer from loneliness, and depression increases.

Stomach problems: Depression can slow down your digestion and cause constipation, reflux, indigestion, and nausea.

Eating disorders: Depression is associated with developing obesity, anorexia, and bulimia.

Chronic pain: Depression plays a part in chronic pain (pain that doesn't go away). Headaches, back pain, muscle aches, joint pain, and chest pain can all be caused by depression. Untreated depression can lead to a life of agony and pain killers. And, guess what? Pain killers can cause or worsen depression. The combination of pain and pain killers could create a vicious cycle that could lead to harmful addictions. If you are suffering from aches and pains with or without a clear cause, consider depression as a contributing factor.

Immune system: Depression weakens the immune system and can cause you to have more colds and flu and to be more susceptible to other diseases.

Sleep disorders: If you are depressed, you may not be able to fall asleep. You may wake in the middle of the night and be unable to fall back to sleep. You may sleep all the time. Or, you may just want to stay in your bed with the shades drawn and the covers over your head. All of these behaviors can be brought on by depression.

Anger and irriatibility: Depression can express itself as anger, frustration, or by being argumentative. These behaviors make relationships very difficult to maintain. People who have closer social relationship and solid marriages live longer and have happier lives than people who are not in happy relationships. Having depression can shorten your life.

Suicide: People who suffer depression tend to have repeated episodes and often the episodes worsen. For some, the depression will progress to the point where the person feels so badly that they believe the only viable option is to take their own life. Up to 70 percent of suicide victims were thought to be depressed at the time of the event.

Depression Assessment Tool

If you have had any of the symptoms listed in the following assessment for more than two weeks, your provider should evaluate you for a diagnosis of depression. In addition to taking the assessment, you may want to read more about depression. It is a problem that is in involved in 80 percent of all primary care visits and is the leading cause of disability in the world.

Depression Assessment

Depression Assessment	Yes	No
Do you have feelings of sadness, isolation, hopelessness, or guilt most of the time? Are people complaining that you are irritable or in a bad mood?		
Do you feel isolated and alone even when people are around?		
Have you lost interest in things that used to bring you joy like hobbies, relationships, sex, or work?		
Are you sleeping too much or too little? Are you tired most of the time?		
Are you having trouble managing your high blood pressure, diabetes, or stomach ailments?		
Do you have unexplained muscle or joint pain, backaches, or headaches?		

Are you eating too much or too little? Do you have a sudden weight gain or loss?		
Are you having thoughts of **suicide?** If so, call your doctor or go to the emergency room and **GET HELP IMMEDIATELY.**		

The answer to "what's causing your problems" may not be in the CAT scan results or the lab test. You may be depressed. Often patients are depressed and providers and patients alike overlook the condition when developing a diagnosis. Yet properly treating depression can make a tremendous difference in the patient's recovery.

Avoid the pitfalls of missing a depression diagnosis. If for any reason you are having trouble managing your disorders; you can't find a clear physical cause for your symptoms; or you have any or all of the symptoms of depression, please be evaluated for depression. If necessary, seek treatment. Depression affects millions of lives and can be a devasting condition. It is not all in your head. It is in your life and your body and help is available.

Your role as team leader:

- **Complete the depression assessment.** If you have had any of the symptoms on the depression assessment for the past two weeks, take this assessment form with you to your provider and have him review it with you.

- **If you feel suicidal, get help immediately.** Call your provider or go to the local emergency room.

- **Get treatment if necessary.** Treatment could save your relationships, your health, your life, or the life of a loved one.

- **Ask for a referral to a therapist or a psychiatrist.** If medication is needed to treat your depression, have an expert manage your medication and seek counseling. Many of the issues that bring about depression are not physical; they are emotional (loss, separation, finacial difficulties, problems with your relationships, and many other things), and you may need help dealing with your issues. You may need a therapist.

- **Don't be ashamed** to say you have depression. Millions of people worldwide are depressed, you are not alone. We are all affected by our emotions and stressful life situations. Don't be ashamed; rather you should seek help.

CHAPTER TEN

You May Need a Second Opinion

"...it is difficult for a specialist to see beyond his own field..."

Joseph A. Jerger, M.D.

Getting a second opinion helps you to confirm or refute a diagnosis, and it enables you to get a different perspective on your treatment options. Dr. B may specialize in treatments of which Doctor A is completely unaware. Dr. A may say the tumor is inoperable, while doctor B may know how to shrink the tumor, thus making it completely operable. There are many clear reasons to get a second opinion. We will discuss those reasons and how to get a second opinion in this chapter.

Reasons to Get a Second Opinion

You are having trouble talking to your doctor

You have not received answers to your questions

You have not received a diagnosis

You are not satisfied with your treatment plan

You're getting worse when you were expecting to get better

You need to have surgery

You're wondering if surgery is your only option

You're going to need a second, unexpected surgery

Your doctor told you no beneficial treatments exist

You have a life-threatening illness. If you have a life-threatening condition, seek the opinion of at least two specialists and compare their opinions and recommendations. Seeking a second or even third opinion for a life-threatening condition is worth the effort. You owe it to yourself to ensure you're getting the best treatment available.

You are diagnosed with a chronic condition. If you are newly-diagnosed with a chronic disease (a disease you are expected to have for a long time) like diabetes, asthma, lupus, arthritis, heart disease, and any other condition that is expected be with you for the rest of your life, ask for a second opinion from a doctor who specializes in your newly-diagnosed condition. A specialist will be able to give you the most up-to-date and specialized care available. When your insurance plan allows for second opinions and specialty care, go for it! You deserve to have expert advice for a condition that is likely to change the way you live your life.

If you have access to providers at a center that specializes in your condition, seek opinions from the professionals at that facility. Not only will the doctors at the specialty center have more experience treating your condition, the center will also employ nursing educators, clinical nurse specialists, nutritionists, and a host of other professionals who are experts in the care you need.

If you are a member of an HMO. Some HMO's have "Gag Rules." A gag rule is a clause written into a provider's contract that forces the provider to keep quiet about methods of care that your insurance policy does not cover or those that are very expensive, even if the more expensive method is better for you. HMO members may not be told of clinical trials or treatments that have only a small chance of success – even if that chance is real – in an attempt to keep down costs. If you are a member of an HMO and you are not satisfied with your treatment plan, you may need a second opinion from an out-of-network provider who is more willing to share information with you.

Probably, I'm not sure, could be, maybe. If you are hearing phrases such as "I'm not sure," "possibly," "probably," or "maybe," you need a second opinion. Yes, medicine is an art and there are a few certainties. However, the provider should have some solid ground to stand on. "Maybe, most likely, and could be" are not enough to make life-changing decisions. Get a second opinion.

The treatment plan seems unusual or wrong. Think of these examples: Your blood pressure is 110/70, normal according to every textbook ever written for an average-sized adult, and the provider suggests you go on blood pressure medication to treat your "pre-high blood pressure." Or, if you have really high blood pressure, 180/110 and the provider says "Let's just wait and see what happens for a couple of weeks." In this case, you could have a stroke in a couple weeks. Get a second opinion.

You live in a poor area. Inner-city Hispanics and Blacks suffer and die at higher than average rates from asthma, diabetes, hypertension, and cancer. If you live in an area with poor outcomes for any disease, get a second opinion from someone who practices outside the area and admits to a hospital where they have better outcomes (you can compare hospitals at (www.hospitalcompare.hhs.gov) outside the area where they have better outcomes.

Your doctor suggested you participate in his clinical trial. If your doctor wants you to participate in a clinical trial on which he is an investigator. Get a second opinion before signing up. It can be hard to find patients to participate in clinical trials and sometimes doctors can be aggressive about recruiting patients for their research projects, even if they don't realize it. A real red flag here is if you are offered incentives to join the clinical trial or the doctor is making you promises about the outcomes.

Your role as team leader:

- **Check with your health insurance carrier.** Learn the procedures for getting in- and out-of-network second opinions. Remember, if you are a member of an HMO and have been diagnosed with a serious condition, you want to seriously consider getting an out-of-network opinion.

- **Ask for a referral to a specialist.**

- **Don't be afraid** you will insult your doctor by asking for names of providers from which you can get a second opinion. Good doctors understand the value of and may even suggest you get a second opinion if she is having difficulty solving a problem. If the provider objects to getting a second opinion in a non-emergent situation, consider this a red flag. Then you should be bold and ask the doctor why she objects.

- **Seek a new perspective.** Doctors who work together in the same practice tend to think alike. Talking to one can be the same as talking to the other one. If you truly want an authentic second opinion, seek a doctor who is not directly associated with the doctor who gave you the first opinion. If two completely separate providers give the same opinion, whether good or bad, it can be reassuring to know you are most likely on the right track. If their opinions differ, you may need a third opinion.

- **Get your records.** Gather all the paper work and test results that relate to your diagnosis. Not having your records will delay care and the provider's ability to offer an opinion based on the facts of your case. Provider B is not going to give her opinion if she does not have your test results. If possible, send your records to the office before the visit. That way, Provider B can review the information before you get to the office. The doctor will thus be more prepared to ask you questions and to offer an opinion.

- **Call your advocate.** Needing a second opinion means something is not quite right. In matters of your health, uncertainty can be very stressful. Your advocate will be able to support you through this stressful time and help you interpret the information you receive during the visit.

- **Get a third opinion if you need one.** It could be possible that the first and second doctors you see will not agree; in fact, they may have very different opinions about what is wrong and what should be done. If this is the case, you may need a third opinion. Keep seeking answers until you feel comfortable with your diagnosis and treatment plan. If you need a third opinion and the insurance company objects or hesitates, you may need to call the case manager to help get the third opinion approved and covered.

Questions to Help You Choose The Best Treatment Option

After you get a second opinion, you may have to decide between two or more treatment options. The following questions will help you to fully evaluate your choices and to make the best decisions.

- **What is the probability of success**?

Ask the doctor how she defines success. Is the treatment going to make your life better? Will it make you worse in any way? Will it prolong your suffering? Can you tolerate the suffering involved? In big treatment decisions, you need these answers.

- **Do you think you can you tolerate the treatment and its side effects?**

Do you want to tolerate the treatment and its side effects, both long- and short-term side effects? Do you want to depend upon a machine or survive with tubes and appliances, (if these things are involved in your treatment)?

- **What will your recovery entail?**

Will you need nursing care at home? Will you need to go to a rehabilitation facility? Will you need someone to drive you around or to shop for you? How will these needs be met?

- **Do you have the support needed for your care?**

Will the insurance company help you find or pay for the care and services you need? Can family members or friends help you or are you alone and unable to manage the plan without support?

- **How far is the treatment from your home?**

Can you travel back and forth by yourself? Who is available to travel with you if you will be sick after the treatment and cannot transport yourself?

- **For each possible choice, ask yourself** "What is the worst thing that can happen?" and If the "worst" does happen, can I live with that?"

Your role as team leader:

- Eliminate options with side effects or outcomes you find unacceptable and do not want to live with.

- Weigh the information and make a decision. If you still aren't 100 percent sure, get additional information from any of the usual sources – the Internet, support groups, and other patients who have had the care you are considering. Ask the provider more questions to clarify any areas you do not fully understand.

- Share your thoughts with your providers and your family. The final treatment decision is yours, but those who love you and have to care for you will be affected by your choices.

- Once you have made your decision, follow through and do what you said you would do. This will give your plan the best chance of success. It is also the best way to build a trusting, working relationship with your provider. You two of you will have a more successful collaboration if you work together openly and honestly.

If You Choose to Do Nothing

If you cannot make a decision, realize that *not* making a decision is the same as making a decision. If you chose to do nothing, you are choosing to "wait and see what happens." This means one of three things:

1. **You may heal spontaneously.** This happens all the time. For example, you have a cold and you don't take any treatment, and you get better on your own. Or, perhaps you have pain and the pain goes away as quickly as it came without any interventions from you or anyone else.

2. **You will get worse** and seeking treatment later will be more complicated or of no use. Generally, the sooner you get proper treatment, the better your chances are of regaining your health.

3. **Choosing no treatment can mean death or disability** will come more quickly than they would with treatment. Not treating out of control blood pressure almost always insures congestive heart failure, a stroke or heart attack will happen in the future.

Of course, sometimes a person chooses no treatment because the treatment itself could shorten their life or affect the quality of their remaining life. In those types of situations, patients have really tough choices to make.

If you come to this point, think about how you want to live the rest of your life. How do you want to feel and what is important to you? Is reading to your children and baking cookies the most important? Is seeking a cure at any cost your goal? Or is your goal something in between? These questions are basically asking "How do you want to live the rest of your life and how do you want to feel while you are living it?" They are quality of life decisions. Think about what you really want and honor yourself.

You may be asking "How will I know what to do?" At some point, you will have to trust the information you have gathered and what one, both, or neither providers has said to you. You will have to trust yourself. Frequently, patients who do not feel right about having a treatment or procedure and end up saving their own lives by refusing care or by choosing a different path. We have all experienced that moment when we said "I should have listened to myself" and the result of not listening was a costly life lesson. Gather and evaluate the facts and then listen to yourself, trust yourself to make a good decision and I wish you and yours all the best.

A Story About Getting A Second Opinion

I was working with a dear friend named Jay in the role of advocate and caregiver for a very serious upcoming back surgery that involved his spinal column. We were facing six to eight hours of surgery and several months of recovery if all went well. If anything went wrong, the possibilities (paralysis, incontinence, pain, and much more) were all bad. We needed to find an excellent orthopedic neurosurgeon. He or she had to be someone we could trust to do a great job and who would be there if we ran into problems after the surgery.

The first surgeon to whom we were referred was a good friend of Jay's primary doctor and was covered under his insurance plan. Let me start by saying we did not like this guy at all. He was arrogant and quite full of both himself and the fact he was a neurosurgeon. Before we began to discuss our case, he had to tell us all about his training and how wonderful he was. When we were "allowed" to speak, the doctor interrupted us to tell us our perceptions and our opinions were wrong.

He could have been super surgeon, at this point it would not have mattered. If we could not talk to him and have our experiences believed and respected, our team could have problems. We needed someone with whom we could work and who would be willing to guide us through care at home.

We finalized the decision not to hire the arrogant doctor based on his lack of experience. He explained he had been to conferences and read the most up-to-date research on our type of case, but had not seen the actual surgery performed in several years. He felt confident, however, that he and his partner could perform the surgery after brushing up on some of the techniques. We were not as sure. Having no experience was clearly unacceptable in a case this complicated. So, we kept looking for Dr. Right.

Something good did happen during that visit. We learned a lot about the different approaches to the surgery and the dangers involved. Dr. Wrong really *had* read up on the problem. He gave us a lot of information, which helped us to talk more confidently to the next provider. We were much more literate and knowledgeable when we left Dr. Wrong's office, and that was a good thing.

We found the surgeon with whom we eventually worked through word-of-mouth. I will call him Dr. Fabulous. He had expert knowledge and a solid history of performing the surgery Jay needed. Of the twelve journal articles in print regarding the surgery, Dr. Fabulous had performed and written about four of them.

His résumé also included being the chief surgeon for two pro sports teams in our state, and he was an excellent educator. He had us make a special appointment so that he could answer all of our remaining questions three days before the surgery. To ensure there was plenty of time for our questions, he booked the visit for 30 minutes.

He gave us a complete overview of the surgery; what it would entail; and what we would need to do at home. He also arranged for us to speak with one of the patients on whom he had performed the surgery Jay was about to undergo. She was very satisfied with her surgical outcome and the care she had received. She highly recommended Dr Fabulous.

We went ahead with the surgery, and needless to say, we had a wonderful outcome. But our wonderful outcome was not magic. We worked for it. We were determined to find the best and safest care available. We learned about the surgery and we had some knowledge of our choices before we met with the surgeons. We asked other providers for advice. We then asked for and received referrals for second and third opinions. We decided together with the doctor on a treatment plan we could live with and the doctor could perform. We took all the steps, suggested in this chapter and it really paid off. I believe we received the best possible care with a great outcome. Today, Jay is pain-free and living a full life, thanks to our hard work and perseverance and because we sought a second opinion and found the best surgeon for the job.

CHAPTER ELEVEN

Preventing Medication Errors

"One of the first duties of the physician is to educate the masses not to take medicine."

William Osler, M.D.

Medication Error: The Facts and Figures

Medication errors occur when doctors are writing prescriptions; when medications are dispensed from the pharmacy; when a healthcare professional or a patient administers the drug; when the drug is monitored for effectiveness; and even when the drug is procured from the manufacturer. Medication errors happen anywhere and everywhere medications are dispensed, and they can happen to anyone at anytime.

According to a July 2006 Institute of Medicine report, medication and prescription errors harm a low estimate of 1.5 million people and take the lives of at least 7,000 patients each year. The study also asserts that many more errors go unreported. The mistakes cost the healthcare system approximately $3.7 billion dollars annually. In this chapter, I will discuss ways in which you can prevent medication errors from happening to you and your loved ones.

Because medication errors occur in both community and hospital settings, I have combined the questions, the reasons why you should ask the questions, and your role as team leader in both environments. I have done this in an attempt to condense the information, and to make it easy to access should you need it in either setting. All of the questions you should ask are contained in the "Questions to Help Prevent Medication and Pharmacy Errors" worksheet in the Appendix and as always hey are there for you to copy and complete as often as like.

Errors at the Pharmacy

A 2003 University of Auburn study predicted the odds of getting a prescription with a serious risk of harm to you as 1 in 1,000. This equates to about 3.7 million pharmacy errors a year based on the number of prescriptions written in 2006.

The large number of prescriptions written every year is a contributing factor to the number of pharmacy errors. In a busy pharmacy, the pharmacist may be required to handle up to 30 prescriptions an hour or one prescription every two minutes. In those two minutes, pharmacists are expected to figure out the doctor's handwriting; check for errors in the prescription; evaluate the new medication for possible drug interactions with your other medications; fill the prescription; and give you counseling and education. They are required to complete these tasks while being constantly interrupted by the phone, technicians needing supervision, and customers needing their help.

In addition to long hours, heavy workloads and constant interruptions, a pharmacist must watch for drugs with similar names, both old and new, that may enter the marketplace at anytime. One in every four medication errors is made because of name confusion. Many drugs have similar names and completely different actions. Drugs such as Cerebyx, Celexa, and Celebrex are each prescribed for very different conditions yet their names are very similar. If you combine the issues of similar drug name and spelling confusion with the problem of poor handwriting, it's easy to see we have a recipe for disaster. Poor handwriting alone puts us all at risk of a medication error and makes you wonder why there are not even more errors.

None of these problems are expected to improve in the near future as the number of prescriptions written each year increases and the number of pharmacists decreases. Between 2004 and 2010, the number of pharmacists is expected to increase by about 8 percent, while the number of prescriptions written is expected to increase by 27 percent. According to the National Association of Chain Drug Stores, in 1994 Americans bought two billion prescriptions. Today, that number has grown to more than three billion and continues to climb.

To meet some of these challenges, pharmacies employ pharmacy assistants and technicians. Requirements vary for technician training from state to state. Depending upon the laws in your state, the technician at your pharmacy could be a high school kid looking for a little pocket money or she could be someone who has attended and successfully completed a formal training program to become a pharmacy technician.

Many technicians, regardless of their level of education are allowed to call doctors and to authorize prescription refills; enter prescriptions into the computer; pull drugs off shelves; and fill prescription bottles. The prescription you recently had filled may have never come into contact with a pharmacist and may have been prepared by a tech who did not understand the drugs being dispensed; their interactions with other drugs; or the decimal points that dictate a proper dosage.

A Story About Decimal Point Error

A mom took her five-year-old son who had a bedwetting problem to the doctor. The doctor prescribed a medication containing 10.0 milligrams of imipramine per teaspoon. The pharmacy tech missed the decimal point and typed in 100 milligrams, ten times the correct amount. The pharmacist did not detect the error and he filled the prescription as the technician had typed it on the label.

The mother gave her little boy the medicine at bedtime as ordered. The next morning, she found her son dead in his bed from a fatal overdose of a prescription medication, caused by an error in the placement of a decimal point. This story is shocking! It is tragic and is reportedly true.

(Source: Consumer.com)

Hospital Medication Errors

Studies indicate that 400,000 preventable drug-related injuries occur each year in hospitals and another 800,000 occur in long-term care settings. Researchers believe that as many as one in every five doses of medication given in a typical hospital or skilled nursing facility is given in error. The average hospitalized patient can expect to experience at least one medication error per day and surgical patients are three times more likely to experience a harmful medication error than patients anywhere else in the healthcare system. Whether you are at your local pharmacy or in the hospital, the most common types of errors (described in detail below) are:

- Lack of informed consent about the drug

- Wrong drug given to the wrong patient

- Wrong dose of the right drug is prescribed

- The wrong method is used to administer the drug (drugs are administered by mouth, IV, injection, inhalation, under the tongue, rectally, vaginally, and through the skin)

- The drug is given at the wrong time

- Omission (the drug was just not given or taken)

Lack of informed consent about medications. By law, providers are required to tell you about the risk and benefits of your medications. You can then decide for yourself if you are willing to take the risks involved with consuming the medication. If a provider does not inform you of the risks and benefits you can reasonably expect to encounter while taking a medication, they are negligent.

In my opinion, lack of informed consent is one of the most serious types of medication errors a prescriber can make. It denies the patient the ability to decide for him or herself if the risks involved in taking a medication are risks they are willing to take. Yet it does not relieve the patient of the consequences of taking the drug should something go wrong. If something does go wrong, the patient pays the price with their health and safety, possibly their life. I don't think that's fair.

Lack of informed consent can have dire consequences. If you do not know you shouldn't drive when starting on a medication because it triggers drowsiness, you may drive right after you take the medication and fall asleep at the wheel. What if you are not told you should avoid a drug while you are trying to get pregnant and your newly conceived child is harmed? These are two of the many dire consequences that result from lack of informed consent.

One of your main goals as the leader of **YOUR** Healthcare Team is to ensure you have informed consent before taking a new medication. To get informed consent, ask these questions:

In the community or the hospital:

Questions to Help Prevent Medication and Pharmacy Errors

- **What is the name of the drug and how do you spell it?**

- **What dose are you prescribing?**

- **Can you write the prescription without decimal points please?** (You want to avoid decimal point confusion whenever possible.)

- **How many times per day should I take the medicine and how many hours apart should I take each dose?** (Does twice a day mean every twelve hours or at 10 a.m. and 6 p.m.? You need to know.)

- **Why am I taking the drug?**

- **What are the side effects of the drug?**

- **What should I do if I develop any of the side effects?**

- **What side effects indicate that I should stop taking the medication?**

- **What side effects indicate that I should call you immediately?**

- **Do I need to avoid any foods, drinks, or activities while on the medication?**

- **Should the medication be taken with food or on an empty stomach?**

- **Does this medication interact with any of my other medications?**

- **Can I just stop taking the drug if it makes me sick?**

- **Is it safe to suddenly stop the medication or does it have to be stopped gradually?**

- **Are there any laboratory tests or self-monitoring activities required while I'm taking this drug?**

For blood pressure medications, you should check your blood pressure periodically, and diabetics should monitor their blood sugars. In addition, many drugs can harm your liver and your kidneys. When taking any of those medications, you will also need to have periodic blood work to assess the health of your vital organs.

- **When should I have lab work done and how often should it be repeated?**

- **How do I perform the monitoring?**

- **Is there anyone who can teach me how to perform the monitoring?**

- **What are the normal results of self-monitoring?**

- **At what point should I call you if my results are abnormal?**

- **How long should I take the drug?**

- **Can I take a generic version of the drug?** (Generic indicates a non-brand name of the drug that is less expensive.)

Dispensing medication to the wrong patient. In this type of error, Mr. I. Jones gets Mr. L. Jones' medication either from a pharmacist or a nurse.

Your role as team leader:
In the community:
- Check the name on your prescription bottles when you receive them from the pharmacist. Read the label and match your pills with the description given on the

information sheet attached to the bag. This way, you will ensure you have the right medication in the bottle.

In the hospital:
- To help prevent the five major categories of medication errors (wrong patient, wrong drug, wrong dose, wrong route, and omission) many hospitals have instituted the "five rights of medication" administration program. In this process the nurse checks that the drug is the right drug, the right dose, given at the right time, and is administered through the right route. Your nurse does these checks outside of your room at the medication cart. After these steps are complete, she comes into the room to identify you and to make sure you are the right person.

This intervention was initiatied because there are many ways and reasons that providers confuse patients in the hospital. And, nurses, the pharmacist, and pharmacy technicians are busy, tired, and over-worked. New orders are written all the time and patients' names sound alike. Technicians can put medications into the wrong patient's drawer, and doctors write orders on the wrong charts. The list of reasons to confuse patients' medications is endless. No matter how many times you are identified, just accept it. Identification is in your best interest as it helps to insure you are the person the nurse intends to give the drug to.

Your role as team leader:

- Do not allow the identification process to be overlooked when you are given your medications in the hospital.

The wrong drug. Two of the biggest reasons patients get the wrong drugs are because of similarly named or packaged medications. For example the pharmacist puts Celexa in the bottle when she should have dispensed Celebrex.

In the community, ask:

- The name of the drug and how the name of the drug is spelled.

- Then, write the name of the drug down on your worksheet as the provider spelled it to compare it later to what the pharmacist has written on your pill bottle.

- What the drug is for and why are you getting it.

- The doctor to email the prescription to the pharmacy or have the medical assistant type out the prescription to avoid problems with understanding the doctor's handwriting.

- Check the medication in the bottle against the description of the medication the pharmacist gives you. A description of the medication can be found on the drug information sheet attached to the package in which the medication is bagged.

In the hospital: In addition to name confusion in the hospital, there can be miscommunication among providers. The doctor could forget to tell the nurse he changed or discontinued a medication and the nurse could give easily give you a cancelled medication. You can help avoid these errors if your doctor tells you about the changes he or she makes to your orders.

Ask:

- All of your providers to inform you of any changes to your medications and ask them what those changes are. Record any changes on your Provider Visit Flow Sheet.

- The nurse to name each of your medications and state their doses to you or your advocate before he or she gives them to you. This way, you can ensure you are getting the right medication and the right dose.

Your role as team leader:

- Know what medications you are taking before you get to the hospital so you do not get the wrong medication(s).

- Inform the staff of any changes that were made to your medication orders before or after your arrival at the hospital, even you think they may already be aware. They may not be aware of every change.

- Take a written list of your medications with you to the hospital.

- Know what the pills you take at home look like. Know how many pills you take and at what time(s) you take them.

- Look at your pills when they are given to you.

- If there are any pills in the little cup you do not recognize, ask what the medication is, who ordered it, how much they ordered it, why they ordered it, when they ordered it, and what its side effects are.

Wrong dosage dispensed. The wrong dosage dispensed occurs in the hospital and the community and it's and easy mistake to make. The prescription reads 10.0 mg and the pharmacy tech puts 100 mg pills in the bottle, ten times the prescribed dose.

Your role as team leader:
- Write down the name of the prescription on your worksheet and read it back to the doctor.

- Read the prescription bottle label and the information

sheet that the pharmacist has attached to the medication. Insure you have the right dose.

- Read the description of the pill on the information sheet and match the medication to its description before you leave the pharmacy.

Wrong route. Drugs are usually given in the form of a pill, liquid, sublingually (under the tongue), by injection, intravenously (IV), suppositories, creams or patches, or by inhaling. If a drug should melt under the tongue and you swallow it whole it may not work the way it's suppose to. It is important that drugs be given by the right route.

In the community ask:
- Your provider for instructions on how the drug should be taken.

In the hospital ask:
- Your provider by which route the drug should be taken.

- Get a print-out of your medication administration sheet from the nurse. The form will include the prescribed route of administration.

Wrong Time. Research shows up to 40 percent of patients have trouble understanding instructions that tell them how to take their medications. Patients confuse things such as taking one pill, two times per day with taking two pills, one time per day. And, many patients have trouble with medical abbreviations. Did you know that "b.i.d." means twice per day at eight-hour intervals, or that "OD" means daily at 10 a.m.? If you answered no, you're not alone. Most people have no idea what these and other abbreviations mean. This is why wrong time is a common type of medication error.

In the community ask:

- The provider at what times and how many times per day you should take the medication. Ask for the answer to be given in plain English; 10 a.m., 2 p.m., and 6 p.m.

- Keep a record of your medications and the times they should be taken.

In the hospital ask:

- The provider or the nurse at what times and how many times per day you should be given the medication.

- Ask for a copy of the medication administration printout, which will include the times your medications are to be given.

- Know what medications and what times you take them at home. If there are changes made at the hospital, ask why those changes were made.

Medication Safety Tips

In addition to the major types of medication errors, others dangers lurk in the land of medication administration. In this section, I will discuss additional measures you can take to be safer when taking your medications. Let's get started.

Research your medication for yourself. Read about your medication, their side effects interactions with your other medications and reasons why patients should not take them on any of the sites listed below or by checking a drug book you can find in any book store or library. By doing a bit of research, you can learn to how to take your medications safely and prevent many common medication errors. When you share what you have learned with your doctor, you will help her to safely prescribe your medications to you. I like the following sites for consumer medication information:

- www.Drugs.com

- www.Walgreens.com

- www.Riteaid.com

- www.Medlineplus.gov

- www.WebMD.com

- www.Mayoclinic.com

Ask the pharmacist about anything you don't understand. Ask anything at all! Ask about the drug's side effects, what to do if you experience side effects, how long to take the drug, and how to take the drug. Ask any questions at all; do not be ashamed to say "I don't understand."

Don't sign anything. Do not sign the sheet at the pharmacy that says you understand how to safely take your medications if you do not fully understand. The register is a legal document. Signing it says the pharmacist gave you informed consent and that all of your questions were answered satisfactorily. Signing that sheet could affect your ability to be compensated if something happens to you or your loved ones because of lack of informed consent.

Review the prescription medications you are taking. At least once a year, bring all of your medicines and supplements with you to each of your providers who prescribe medication. During the visit, discuss your medications and ensure you are taking the right combination of drugs. You and your providers can also decide if you need to make any changes. Ask your doctors if any of your medications are unnecessary duplications or if any of them could be interacting with one another.

Tell your doctor about the supplements, over-the-counter

drugs, and natural therapies you use. Did you know Motrin (ibuprophen), St. John's Wort, Ginkgo Balboa, Vitamin A and E can all prolong bleeding time? All of these products, therefore, should be stopped days before any scheduled surgery. If they are not stopped they could contribute to a hemorrhage during or after the operation.

My point is this: Tell your doctor about the supplements you take and research the side effects and interactions for yourself. Your doctor may not know supplement side effects because most doctors have no training in natural therapies. By researching your supplements you will help your doctors prescribe conventional medications in a safer fashion.

Take drugs that have been on the market for a long time. A drug could be on the market for several years before we discover it has devastating side effects. Despite the best efforts of the FDA and others to ensure drug safety, every year drugs are recalled that were once thought to be safe. We find out a drug is not safe only after several people have been hurt, or when a major class action suits is initiated to collect damages for those the medication has injured. You don't want to be a patient hurt by a new drug. Whenever possible, take drugs that have been proven over time to be safe and effective. Do not rush to take the latest and the greatest drug if you have an older, safer, and cheaper option.

Report all allergies and drug reactions to the provider immediately. If you become red and itchy; if you break out in a rash; or you have difficulty breathing you are having an allergic reaction. Report this right away. Meet your provider at the emergency room, because allergic reactions are life threatening!

Report side effects. Sometimes you can't take your medications because they cause side effects you find unacceptable. Don't just stop the medication without telling your doctor and giving her the opportunity to safely make adjustments to your regimen. Some drugs need to be stopped slowly and others may need to have their dose adjusted or completely changed. Work with your physician to find the right medication and right dose.

If your medication requires a special device or measuring instrument, be sure you know how to use it. Not knowing how to use the medication could be deadly. I have seen patients come into the hospital having a full-blown asthma attack because they were never taught how to properly use the inhaler used to administer their asthma medication. If you have questions about how to use a device or how to measure your medications, ask the office nurse, the pharmacist, or the nurse at the hospital to teach you how to use the device or equipment. If you still have questions, call the device's manufacturer to get instructions directly from a company representative.

Store and handle medications properly. Medications may need to be refrigerated or stored in a dark place. Some should not be handled with bare hands or by women who are pregnant or may become pregnant. Medications expire and need to be disposed of after they expire. Find out if there is any special storage or handling requirements for your medications. Follow those instructions to keep you and your family safe.

Be careful and use your medications safely. During the time I was writing this book, Michael Jackson, Anna-Nicole Smith, and Heath Ledger all passed away. Each of their deaths involved using multiple medications simultaneously. In the case of Mr. Ledger, he was reportedly a victim of an accidental overdose of Valium, Temazepam, and Xanax (three anti-anxiety drugs); Vicodin and Oxycodone (two pain medications); and Unisom, a sleeping medication. Any two of those medications in any combination could be life threatening. There are (were) reportedly several doctors under investigation for writing those prescriptions. However, Mr. Ledger may have been the only one who knew everything he was taking. He, therefore, was the only person who could have kept himself safe from the effects of combining all of those drugs. It behooves each of us to know the risks, benefits, interactions, and contraindications (reasons not to take) of all the drugs you are taking. As we used to say when I was growing up. "You better check yourself, before you wreck yourself!!"

CHAPTER TWELVE

Hospital Errors and How to Avoid Them

"Prepare and prevent, don't repair and repent."
Unknown

The Facts and Figures

HealthGrades Incorporated, our nation's leading healthcare ratings organization reviewed the records of 40 million hospitalized Medicare patients (patients aged 65 and older) between the years of 2002-04. The investigators were looking for evidence of 16 types of patient safety incidences (medical errors). They choose this group of errors to investigate because they were deemed suitable for administrative review by the Agency for Healthcare Research and Quality and because specific measures could be put into place to track them. The study revealed the following information:

- There were 1.24 million patient safety incidences in our nations hospitals associated with the 16 types of errors.

- The number of errors increased by nearly 9 percent since the previous study.

- Six types of errors worsened by nearly 12 percent since the previous study.

- Over the three-year period, 304,702 senior citizens died after falling victim to multiple hospital errors

- The errors generated 9.3 billion dollars in excess Medicare costs.

Additionally, a group of hospital errors known as "never events" has recently gained a good deal of attention because they happen regularly to hospitalized patients and because they are responsible for billions in excess healthcare costs. The comprehensive list of never events includes:

- Death or serious disability associated with a medication

- Infections from intravenous and central lines

- Development of a stage three or four pressure ulcer (a really bad bedsore) after being admitted to a healthcare facility

- Death or serious disability associated with a blood transfusion

- Death or serious disability associated with intravascular air embolism

- Surgery performed on the wrong body part

- Surgery performed on the wrong patient

- Wrong surgical procedure performed

- Leaving behind foreign objects in a patient after surgery or other procedure

- Intra-operative or immediately post-operative death in a low-risk patient This means that the patient was basically healthy when he or she was admitted to the hospital and there was no expectation the patient would die as a result of the surgery

- Death or serious disability associated with hypoglycemia (really low blood sugar)

- Death or serious disability associated with a fall

- Death or serious disability associated with an electric shock

- Maternal death or serious disability associated with labor or delivery in a low-risk mother

- Infants discharged to the wrong person.

- Death or serious disability associated with failure to identify and treat hyperbilirubinemia (jaundice) in newborns.

Failure to rescue, with an incidence rate of 155 per every 1,000 patients is the largest category of hospital error. This category includes failure to diagnose and/or treat a problem in time to prevent an injury and inappropriate or substandard treatment (negligence). The aforementioned both lead to a hospitals' failure to prevent a patient from becoming worse while in their care and belong to the category of error known as "failure to rescue".

Let's look at an example of failure to rescue and getting worse while in the care of the hospital. Let's say you go to the hospital with really high blood sugars, (heaven forbid, but let's just pretend). The doctor orders insulin, and that's were the trouble begins. When your nurse comes to check on you and you appear to be sleeping. She fails to realize you have slipped into a coma because of your very low blood sugar. When your condition is discovered you are rushed to ICU in the hopes of preventing permanent injury and death. This is an example of failure to rescue, diagnose, and treat in time, and this type of error is an all-too common occurrence in hospitals.

The good news from the HealthGrades study is that

250,246 or 82 percent of the found errors could have been prevented. That means that you and your team members have the potential to prevent hospital errors from happening to you and your loved ones as well.

In this chapter, I discuss several types of hospital error and what you can do to decrease your chances of becoming a victim of them.

Choose A Good Hospital

The first thing you should do to ensure your safety while in the hospital is to choose a good hospital to be admitted to. The top 15 percent of hospitals in the United States significantly outperformed the bottom 15 percent in each of the never event categories and in overall patient safety. The superior performance of these hospitals results in patients having a 43 percent lower risk of falling victim to a medical error while in their care. If all hospitals performed at the level of those distinguished for patient safety, there would have been 44,153 fewer deaths in the Healthgrades study and $2.45 billion dollars saved during 2002-04. Therefore I say, one of most important things you can do to prevent a hospital error is to choose one of the safest hospitals for the care of your illness and have your treatment in that facility. Here's what you need to know to do just that.

Teaching hospitals do a little worse than non-teaching

hospitals in terms of error, and hospitals that specialize in a particular type of care tend to have better outcomes in their area of specialty than hospitals that do not specialize. Generally speaking the best care for cancer will be found at a cancer center and the best care for a transplant will be found at a facility that specializes in the care of transplants patients and so on. You can find out how the hospital to which you want to be admitted is rated in comparison to other hospitals in your area by researching your choices at one of the following sites:

- www.HealthGrades.com

- www.JCAHO.org

- www.Healthfinder.com

- www.hospitalcompare.hhs.gov

During the investigative process you should ask yourself and find answers to the following questions.

Questions to Help You Choose the Best Hospital

- **Does the hospital specialize in treating my condition?**

- **If not does the hospital care for a lot of people with my condition?**

The more experience a hospital has with a condition, the better their performance record in the treatment of that condition will be.

- **How does the hospital compare with others in my area?**

You will find this answer at www.hospitalcompare.hhs.gov. This site rates hospitals in multiple areas including infections rates and the care of specific diseases and compares their performance with other hospitals.

- **Is this hospital covered by my health insurance?**

If a hospital is not covered by your plan and you need specialized care that can only be given at that hospital, call your insurance carrier. Ask to speak to the case manager who can perhaps negotiate a contract with the hospital for your care.

- **Does my clinician have privileges; that is, is she allowed to work at the hospital?**

Often doctors have privileges at more than one hospital, yet they may prefer to work at one hospital rather than another. Ask your doctor if she has privileges at the hospital of your choice, even if she routinely practices at another facility.

General Hospital Safety

After you are admitted to the hospital, the work for you and your advocate really begins. In this section, I will discuss things you and your advocate need to do to stay safe while you are in the hospital. Some of the measures listed below are agreed upon by experts and are taken right out of the latest literature. Some of the measures suggested in this section are based upon what I have seen, done, experienced, and taught patients over the last two decades.

Don't go near a teaching hospital in July if you can help it. If you are having an elective procedure (something that is not an emergency and you have time to plan), July may not be a good time to have that procedure done. Medical students, interns, and new residents traditionally start their training on July 1st. New nurses who have just graduated and passed their board exams also start their first jobs in July. To avoid the chaos, many seasoned professionals go on vacation during this time, leaving the hospital filled with new people trying to learn their jobs and find their way around. If you can avoid teaching hospitals until everyone gets their bearings, it will be better for you. In my experience, things start to settle down around September.

Go to the hospital with your advocate. It is my belief

and the experts agree that everyone who enters the hospital needs an advocate at his or her side. If you have been in the hospital lately, you have experienced how chaotic they can be. There are lots people in and out of the patients' room on any given day; dietary, housekeeping, social workers, case managers, therapists, nurses, physicians, specialty physicians, interns, and residents will enter a patient's room. On a single hospital admission, a patient can expect to meet up to 100 new people. Just to complicate matters, the staff and team members change frequently. Nurses often work 12-hour shifts, which means they work three days per week and have vacations and holidays in between. Doctors go on vacation and are "covered" by colleagues. Residents and interns switch rotations or cover for one another. Amidst all of these changes are many opportunities for information to be lost or distorted as it is reported (or not reported) from one person to the other.

Your advocate can be the team member who manages your health history and the history of your hospitalization. Your advocate can communicate with other team members and tell them what happened last night or the night before. They can let team members know what Dr. So and So said about this or that. Advocates are able to help prevent medication errors when they are familiar with you and the medications you are taking. Some of the other great things that advocate do are to:

- Let providers know how well treatments are working or not working

- Monitor you for side effects and reactions to medications

- Call for help when needed

- Provide personal care the nurses can't provide because of time constraints and short staffing.

- A good advocate is an invaluable asset to you while you are in the hospital.

Note: If your advocate likes to argue or is inconsiderate of other team members, you may want to rethink who your hospital advocate will be. An argumentative advocate could make members of **YOUR** Healthcare Team want to avoid your room while he or she is around and that's not good. Try to choose an advocate who "plays well with others," even when they feel like screaming and who can remember that it's nice to be nice.

There is one last thing I would like to say in tis section before I move on; and that is "Thank You!," to every good advocate out there helping and protecting their loved ones when they need them the most. We are all better off because of you and what you do, so again I say, a heartfelt thank you.

Bring a copy of your healthcare proxy and living will. Have copies of your healthcare proxy and living will placed in your chart and made part of your medical record and identify your advocate/proxy as the person who will speak for you should the need arise. Identifying your advocate early in the hospitalization will let the other team members know they can speak freely to your advocate and share information with her. This will facilitate communication throughout your hospital stay, especially in case of an emergency when your advocate may need to give information or permission for treatments.

Bring your Provider Visit Flow Sheet with you. You can greatly enhance your safety while you are in the hospital by recording all of the communication that occurs around you and your care. When you keep track of your orders for tests, medications, and treatments, you will ensure accurate communication among all members of your team. To perform this function, you or your advocate should use the Provider Visit Flow Sheet to record any new medications that are ordered and by whom; medications that were changed in dosage or discontinued; and any testing or procedures that were ordered or cancelled. Having this information will help you and your advocate coordinate your care and prevent the errors that occur because of poor communication between other members of your team.

Bring this workbook with you and get fully informed consent. Any time anyone suggests a test, procedure, or surgery you need informed consent. Take the "Questions To Help You Understand Your Diagnosis and Treatment Options" worksheet with you and ask the questions it contains. This will help you get fully informed consent before agreeing to any treatments or procedures.

Identify a point person. There are frequently situations in the hospital where Dr. A is waiting for Dr. B; Dr. C is covering for Dr. D; and none of your doctors know exactly what's going on. You may not have any idea what is supposed to happen next. You may not know when or if you are being discharged or if you are going for another CAT scan in the morning. Nurse case managers and nurses are the team members responsible for knowing all of that information and for the coordination of your care plan. Case managers in a coordination role talk to all of your doctors and relay information among them, to other team members, and to you. Case managers help ensure the exchange of information and decrease treatment delays that occur because of poor communication. Ask to speak with the case manager assigned to coordinate your care your care and maintain an open line of communication with her. Ask her to keep you and your advocate informed of her findings.

Nurse as case manager. Nurses are responsible for knowing where you are, what test and procedures you are scheduled, if surgery is planned or cancelled, your diet, physical therapy and much more. When the nurse knows what is happening or not happening, she can prevent tests and procedures that were scheduled in error; block wrong medications; and prevent many other adverse events. However, coordinating the care of several patients is a very complicated task. Your nurse may have up to eight patients for whom she is responsible. Each patient may have four or five doctors, multiple diagnosis, and several treatment plans. Trying to keep up with all of that in an environment where people from different disciplines and departments may not be talking to one another is very difficult. This is why your nurse needs your help to help keep you safe. You or your advocate should keep your nurse in the loop. Let her know what Dr. So and So said the plan is for tomorrow is and what your responses to treatments have been. Tell her what happened when you went downstairs for testing. Share with her any information about your care that she was not present to witness for herself. Do not assume she knows what is happening. Unfortunately, you cannot assume the members of your team are talking to one another. The information you share will help your nurses to keep you safe.

Tell your nurses your story. Tell your nurse the history of the illness that brought you to the hospital and the effects it has had upon you and your family. Help her to understand you and connect with you as a person. Use the O.L.D.C.A.R.T.S format to tell the nurse what you have experienced – both the good and the bad. Let the nurse know anything outside of your medical diagnosis that may be affecting you. If you have not heard from one of your children in days and you are a nervous wreck, let the nurse know. Your emotional state affects your responses to treatment and your healing. Knowing what is going on with you helps the nurse connect with you and care for you as a person, not just a patient. Her caring makes her a stronger advocate for you. Moreover, her advocacy could help to save your life.

Be nice to your nurse. When you are nice to your nurses, you are more likely to be treated with an extra level of respect and kindness and that will go a long way toward enhancing your safety. Just saying "thank you" and "please" helps build a positive relationship between you and your nurse in which you both feel comfortable sharing information.

Bring stuff. Nurses love it when patients bring them gifts. If you or your family members bring gifts, you will be moved up to favorite patient status. Your kindness will most likely be repaid with extra time and attention. Bring bagels, doughnuts, fruit, pizza, candy, flowers, whatever you like. Anything you bring is an investment in your safety.

Notify staff before you need them. Try to call for your nurse before your need becomes urgent. When you notice your IV bag has about two inches of fluid left, call the nurse. Leave time for him to respond before the bag is completely empty. Call the nurse for pain medication when the pain starts; don't wait until it gets really bad. Invariably it will take the nurse time to bring medication and the pain could be much worse by the time you're your nurse gets around to delivering you your medication. Likewise, if you need help going to the bathroom, don't wait until the last minute because it does take time for help to arrive. This is especially true when shift changes occur, typically between 7 a.m. and 8 a.m.; 3 p.m. and 4 p.m.; again at 7 p.m. and 8 p.m.; and between 11 p.m. and midnight. It may be difficult to get any help as the day shift leaves and the night shift comes in because the entire staff is "in report." Ask for help before your condition becomes urgent, and try to call for help before or after shift change if it at all possible.

Monitor medication reactions. If you think you are having a bad reaction to any new medication, let your nurse know right away! Refuse to take repeat doses of the medication until you get clarification about what happened and you are sure it is safe to continue taking the medication. Better safe than sorry. New medications, especially IV medications, can cause rapid changes that may go unnoticed. You and your advocate should monitor your reactions to anything you are given and report distress or unexpected side effects to the nurse immediately.

Ask family and friends to stop by. Nurses tend to be more attentive to patients who have the most visitors. Having visitors makes you more attractive and it lets staff know you are being looked after by loved ones.

When you have a complaint. When you have a complaint, your first course of action should be to discuss the circumstances of your complaint with the people involved and make them aware of your concerns. If after you discuss your problem it is still not resolved, you may want to call the patient representative. Patient representatives have a wide and varied role in assuring patient satisfaction. In addition to trying to help settle disputes, they can help you with filling out and signing healthcare proxies; they can arrange for transportation and translation services; and help find lost items. If you want to transfer to another hospital or if you want to fire your doctor and need to find another one while in the hospital, it is the patient representative's job to help you do all of these things and more. If there are problems the patient representative cannot resolve, contact the nurse manager of your unit. If it is a weekend and the manager is not working, contact the nursing supervisor. If there is no help for you down either of those avenues, call the hospital administrator on duty to get help with your problem. Let the staff know you will not suffer poor treatment and that you will call for assistance with conflict resolution when you need it.

Hospital Infections and How to Avoid Them.

One in every 20 hospitalized patients will develop an infection from something to which they were exposed in the hospital: an IV, a surgical wound, a urinary catheter, a procedure, or an infected and contagious roommate are all among the many causes of hospital-acquired infections. Hospital-acquired infections may lead to weeks of hospitalization, trips to the ICU, the loss of limbs, and/or death. These deadly infections took the lives of 90,000 patients in 2002, and they cost our healthcare system more than $30 billion dollars per year to treat. In this section, I will discuss ways you can help prevent a hospital-acquired infection.

Your Role as Team Leader:
Number one rule: Wash your hands! Hand washing is an important way to prevent the spread of infections. Yet, it is not done regularly or thoroughly enough. When you are in the hospital and you notice someone is about to touch you who has not washed his or her hands, ask that person to do so. It will make a difference. A recent study found that when

patients ask their team members if they had washed their hands, the team members washed their hands more often and used more soap.

Wash your hands too. You and family members should wash your hands too. You touch your own wounds, you put food in your mouth. You may have bacteria and even super bacteria all over you after a few days in the hospital. Keep sanitary wipes and/or a hand sanitizer by your bed and use them to clean your hands. This is especially important if you are confined to bed and have to use a bedpan. Your hands will become soiled and it is possible you will not be offered a washcloth to clean them. You can ask the staff for wipes and hand sanitzers as well, if they are not supplied, be prepared to bring your own.

Talk to housekeeping about cleaning everything. Do you know what the most contaminated part of a hospital room is? It's the TV remote control (which is often the nurse call bell too). This device lies in the bed with patients who have any number of infectious conditions; it is one of the most-touched objects in any hospital room; and it is one of the least cleaned objects. To help decrease your chances of becoming infected, ask the housekeeping staff to use a new disposable cloth for each part of your room, including the remote control, the bathroom, the bed, and the furniture. Each of these objects needs its' own cleaning cloth. Ask the housekeeper to use the spray cleaner/disinfectant in your room and not water from a common bucket that he or she has used to clean other rooms.

Monitor your area for infectious objects. Hospital rooms are small and have little countertop space to store things. Nurses and techs sometimes put urinals, (urine containers) on the patient's bedside stand. This is the same stand where your dinner tray will be placed, and the same bedside stand where bandages and dressings will be prepared to put on your open surgical wound.

Do not allow unclean objects to be placed on your bedside stand or on any surface providers use to prepare equipment for dressing changes or other procedures. Ask nurses and physicians who perform dressing changes or procedures at your bedside to wipe the stand (where they prepare their equipment and place them on the stand) with alcohol before they open clean supplies.

Ask your doctor if you really need that antibiotic. Antibiotics are a huge part of hospital-acquired infections. Antibiotics kill both good and bad bacteria and in doing so they disrupt your body's natural defenses (you need the good bacteria to keep you healthy). Antibiotics can cause the bad bacteria, such as Clostridium Difficile, to overgrow and cause you to develop painful diarrhea or worse. Clostridium Difficile, commonly known as C-Diff, is a serious infection and it comes about because of use and overuse of antibiotics.

Sometimes doctors give antibiotics to prevent an infection that you do not have. This could be either dangerous or it could be really necessary. Ask if you really need that antibiotic and how soon it can be discontinued if you do really need it.

Ask for Acidophilus. Acidophilus, the culture in yogurt, promotes intestinal health by keeping the good and the bad bacteria in balance. In doing so it can help prevent the development of a hospital acquired infection associated with over use of antibiotics. Studies have shown acidophilus to be a safe and cost-effective way to boost your immunity and help your body protect itself from the ill effects of over using antibiotics. It will also help you digest and eliminate food. Anytime you are prescribed an antibiotic, ask the provider to order acidophilus at the same time.

Ask your doctor if you really need that antacid. Often patients are given Pepcid, Nexium, or some other gastric secretion-blocking drug while in the hospital. This is done because being in the hospital is stressful and can cause patients to develop ulcers. It is also thought that some of the drug combinations patients take while in the hospital can cause ulcers as well. To prevent these conditions, doctors prescribe acid-blocking drugs. Here's the problem. Your gastric acid accounts for approximately 70 percent of your immune function. If you do not have gastric acid, you loose your first line of immunity, which is not the best thing in an environment where infection runs rampant. If you are not suffering gastric upset or any condition for which you really need antacids, ask why you need them. If the reasoning is not sound, you may want to refuse the medication, because decreasing gastric acid with acid-blocking drugs means decreasing your natural immunity.

Eat right. Unfortunately eating right may mean avoiding a lot of the hospital's food. Take foods (and I use the word loosely here) like Jell-O. Jell-O is food coloring, sugar, and fat. Need I say more? You are sick, weak, just had surgery, been in an accident, have cancer, or any number of other things that have made you sick enough to go to the hospital, and the hospital feeds you red, sugary fat. As if that wasn't bad enough sugar decreases the functioning of your immune system. Sugary foods should not be a part of any healing diet. So then the question becomes, what do you eat? Here are some answers.

If you are on clear liquids, ask if your family can bring vegetable broth, chicken broth, and apple juice. Drink green tea because it has antioxidants that will help you fight infection.

While on full liquids, you can also drink Miso, a soy protein soup. Protein helps repair and build new tissue. Ask your loved ones to bring you fruit and vegetable smoothies (again, fruits and vegetables help boost your immunity). Eat plenty of oranges, grapefruit, lemons, and apples and drink their juices. Pomegranate, and blueberry juices are powerful antioxidants, which also boost immune function and a splash of grape juice will also help boost the spirits. Drinking plenty of water and fruit juices promotes healthy elimination. Whenever you clean the body of toxins and decrease your risk of infection and you are healthier because of it.

Get Out of Bed!! If you can. When lying in the bed for long periods of time your lungs do not fully expand. Fluid and bacteria can build up in the lungs and cause pneumonia to develop. By getting out of bed, you will cause your lungs to expand and that will help remove old fluid and prevent new fluid from collecting. By moving around, you increase your circulation and help prevent blood clots from forming and causing their own life-threating issues. (Blood clots are a major cause of death in hospitalized patients.) It is very important that you get out of bed as soon as possible! If you need help moving, ask for help from physical therapy and the nursing attendants – whatever you need – just move, if you can.

Don't cover your mouth when you cough or sneeze!! We have all been taught to cover our mouths when we cough. We were all taught incorrectly!! When you sneeze or cough into your hands, you expel mucus and germs onto them. Afterward, you touch your IV lines, your dressings, your food, your pen, your table, your eyes, your loved ones, the computer, and the phone – all while your hands are covered in recently expelled germs. We all say we wash our hands after we cough and sneeze, but do we really leave our desks or our phone conversations after we sneeze to wash our hands? Can you wash your hands after you sneeze if you are confined to a bed? No, of course not.

So what should you do? The answer is to cough or sneeze to the floor. Put your head down beside your knees if you are sitting so you don't spray anyone, including yourself. Using this method of expulsion, you never touch the infected spray of mucus and saliva. The heavy droplets filled with germs, mucus, and saliva fall to the floor and die and that is the end of them; that is, unless someone goes down on the floor and gets them. In that case, I think the person who gets them off the floor should have them!

Further, when you sneeze or cough in your hands, you can prolong the life of a cold by up to three days. If you do not cough or sneeze in your hand, you can shorten the cold and decrease the spread of germs to yourself and others. Just in case you're wondering, I have been teaching this for 13 years and sneezing to the floor even longer than I have been teaching. I have *never* sprayed anyone or talked to anyone else who has.

Decubitus Ulcers/Pressure Ulcers/ Bedsores and How to Prevent Them

Decubitus ulcers, also known as pressure ulcers and bedsores, are recorded as occurring in 33 out of 1,000 hospital admissions. This result reflects a 9 percent increase from previous studies. A pressure ulcer is the breakdown of your skin and muscles that can cause a gapping hole to develop where your muscle tissue used to be. In the most severe cases, patients are unable to walk or sit up in a chair (possibly ever again) because of the lost muscle mass. Pressure ulcers represent a loss of mobility, possible infections, surgeries and a good deal of pain and suffering. These ulcers are very serious and, of course, cost thousands and thousands of dollars to treat. They are also included in the group of diagnosis known as never events, which makes them a diagnosis Medicare and many others will not pay to treat. In Medicare's opinion, the ulcer should have never happened, so they are not willing to pay for its' treatment. What does this mean for the patient with the decubitus ulcer? It likely means treatment needed for a pressure ulcer once the patient leaves the hospital will not be covered by thier insurance company. The care of decubitus ulcers could include antibiotics, physical therapy, or surgery and they could bankrupt the average American family. It is very important to prevent these horrible, painful ulcers from occurring to you or your loved ones. Here's how.

Your role as team leader:

Turn every two hours: Because decubitus ulcers are caused by prolonged pressure on a weakened or vulnerable body part, they may be prevented by changing the patient's position every two hours and relieving the pressure that causes them. Patients should be turned or repositioned in bed every two hours to relieve areas of pressure where the weight of the body promotes skin breakdown.

Form a partnership with the nursing staff. Ask your nurses everyday to check your vunerable areas for evidence of redness or broken skin. Red sore spots are also known as stage one ulcers (the stages are 1-4) and could be the start of big trouble. The progression of stage one ulcers can also be halted, however, before they cause any real problem.

Make sure your loved one is clean and dry. Ask the nurses to check your incontinent loved ones every two hours for evidence of soiling. In addition to washing the area during each changing, have the staff use a moisturizing barrier cream to protect the skin. This will add a level protection from the irritants contained in waste products and help heal any minor damage that has already been done. Massage the skin while applying moisturizing agents to enhance blood flow and the growth of healthy skin.

Hospital safety requires that you and your advocate are diligent and your safety is worth all the effort.

CHAPTER THIRTEEN

Surgical Errors and How to Prevent Them

"I can assure you these numbers are just the tip of the iceberg."
Dennis O'Leary, Director Joint Commission

Surgical Dangers: The Facts and Figures

As with any category of error, it is impossible to know exactly how many surgical errors actually occur every year. The rate of wrong site surgery is reported as 1 in 112,994 operations. A review conducted at the University of Washington Hospital found instruments were left in one of every 5,000-20,000 surgical patients or about two to three times a year at that hospital. Again, no one knows how often instruments are left in patients, because no one routinely collects data in this area. Dennis O'Leary, head of the Joint Commission, which inspects more than 18,000 hospitals and surgical centers nationwide, said "I can assure you the numbers are just the tip of the iceberg. Some hospitals are reporting everything and some hospitals are not reporting anything." However, we do know, based upon a study that reviewed 15,000 medical records in Colorado and Utah, that 54 percent of surgical errors are preventable.

In 2001, the Joint Commission sounded an alarm among healthcare professionals to correct surgical errors, without much improvement. Out of frustration, the Joint Commission later said the best way for things to get better is to get patients involved. Getting involved means, in part, getting fully informed consent about your surgery before deciding to have it, and then choosing the best surgeon and hospital for your care. The following questions and information will help you to do just that.

Questions to Help You Get Fully Informed Surgical Consent

- **Why do I need surgery?**

- **Is there some other way to treat my condition?**

- **What kind of surgery do I need?**

- **What will you be doing while inside me? How will you rearrange my parts?**

- **What will my body look like after the surgery?**

- What are the benefits and risks of having this surgery?

- Will the surgery make my life better and for how long?

- Will the surgery make my life worse and for how long?

- How many times have you done this surgery?

- What do you consider a successful surgery?

- How often is this surgery successful?

- Is there another surgical procedure from which I can choose?

- What are the risks and benefits of the other option?

- What will happen if I wait or do not have this surgery?

- How much will it hurt and how do you or the pain management team plan to control my pain?

- Will I need general anesthesia?

- Can I have something other than general anesthesia?

One of the largest areas of malpractice is anesthesia, because anesthesia is a major cause of surgical complications and death. If you can have regional or local anesthesia, it could be a better choice.

- **How long will the surgery take?**

This speaks to how much time you will spend under anesthesia and how much risk you face because of it. If you have heart, lung, kidney, or liver problems that prevent drugs from being eliminated from your body, the amount of time you are under anesthesia is an important safety consideration. If you have any of these problems ask your anesthesiologist how they will affect your care, and how he plans to monitor your safety.

- **Will I wake up with any tubes, drains, or special equipment attached to me?**

You don't want to be surprised by machines and monitors when you wake up. You would rather know in what condition you will wake up before hand so that you and your advocate will not be surprised or unduly stressed by unexpected events.

- **How long will I have this equipment?**

- **Will someone teach me how to care for my tubes, drains, and bandages?**

- **How long will it take for me to recover?**

- **Will I need to spend time in a rehabilitation center?**

- **How long will I be in the hospital?**

- **How much will the surgery cost?**

- **Will my health insurance cover the surgery?**

- **Where can I get a second opinion?**

Getting a second opinion is highly recommended anytime surgery is suggested. See the section on how to get a second opinion to help guide you through this process.

Questions to Help You Choose the Best Surgeon and Hospital for Your Surgery

- **What are the doctor's qualifications to perform this surgery?**

Board certified surgeons have completed many extra hours of training in their area of specialty and passed written examinations to earn the title "board certified." Ask your surgeon if he is board certified in the type of surgery he is suggesting you have. If he is not you may want to find one who is. Some surgeons have F.A.C.S. after their name. This means they are a Fellow in the American College of Surgeons and have passed an even higher level of review by top members of their profession.

- **How much experience do you have doing this operation?**

One way to reduce the risks of surgery is to choose a surgeon who has been well trained and has plenty of experience performing the operation. Ask your surgeon how many times he or she has performed the surgery under consideration and about his recent record of success and complications. Ask how his other patients doing after the surgery? Ask if you can talk to them and hear their stories for yourself.

- **Who will assist you? How well trained is that person?**

- **At which hospital will the operation be done?**

Your surgeons may work at more than one hospital. Find out at which hospital your doctor prefers to work at and how often the same operation is done there.

- **What is the success rate at each of the hospitals?**

If your surgeon suggests using a hospital with a lower success rate for your surgery, find out why. Maybe hospital B gives more personalized care and has fewer infections and a really good rehabilitation doctor. Ask why the doctor would choose one hospital over another and weigh your options and don't forget to compare hospital performances at www. hospitalcompare.hhs.gov.

How To Be Safer During Surgery

There are many things that can go wrong during the surgical process and things you can do to enhance your safety. Let's look at some of the most common types of surgical errors and what you can do to prevent them from happening to you and your loved ones. Some of the most common types of surgical errors are:

- Surgery on the wrong patient

- Surgery on the wrong body part

- Leaving a surgical instrument, sponge, or needle inside of a patient

- Failure to stop medications that can cause injury or death (before, during or after) the surgery

- Unexpected death of an otherwise healthy patient

during the surgical process or immediately following the operation

Your role as team leader:

- **Review your medications with the surgeon and the anesthesiologist.** Make a special request to have the surgeon and the anesthesiologist or their assigns review your medications with you 72 hours before surgery. Medications that cause bleeding such as Plavix or Coumadin, Aspirin, Motrin, Ginkgo, Vitamin E, and blood sugar lowering medications may need to be stopped, adjusted, or monitored well in advance of the surgery.

- **Ask if the hospital performs instrument counts. If not, ask if they would for you.** Some hospitals count all instruments; some only count needles and sponges; however instruments, sponges and needles are left behind during surgery. Ask to have the team members count needles, sponges and instruments. If the surgeon is not willing or does not know how to arrange these counts call the nurse manager of the operating room and ask her, to facilitate your request.

- **Mark the body part on which you are having surgery to prevent having the wrong body part operated on.** Use an indelible marker to write your name and something indicating this is the right spot.

- **Mark the opposite side body part "wrong site" or "not here."** Both sides need to be marked. If the surgeon looks at only the wrong site, he may not expose the correct site and could miss the marking on the right site completely.

- **Mark the surgical site with your name.** Have the nurse identify you out loud. The nurse should identify you by name, date of birth, and social security number immediately prior to the surgery. He should also confirm the type of surgery you are having before you enter the actual operating room.

- **Remind your surgical team to take a time out**. A time out is a process in which the team members pause before an incision is made to discuss the case. They should identify the patient one last time and review films to ensure they are operating on the correct body part and the correct side of the body. Talk this over with the surgeon before hand, especially if this is not standard procedure, so that he can arrange with team members to get needed films and scans prior to your arrival in the operating room. Not all teams take a time out, but this measure has been shown to reduce surgical errors and to improve patient safety, so it's well worth the effort.

- **Take a "prepare for surgery" course**. There are courses you can take prior to surgery to prepare you for the procedure. These courses promote healing through visualization and meditation and the research findings on patients who have taken these courses is amazing. Patients who took the Peggy Huddleston Heal Faster program reported up to 50 percent less pain after knee and hip replacement than patients who did not take the class. In many cases, patients who took the course left the hospital a day earlier, were able to move better, and had better digestion after their surgeries as well. You can find out how to take the Peggy Huddleston course in the privacy of your own home by visiting www.healfaster. com. I have used this program with patients and achieved excellent results. Of course, there are other programs to choose from. Look around and find the course that works best for you. Good luck with your surgery! I wish you all the best.

Chapter Fourteen:

You Need Good Discharge Instructions

"Education is not preparation for life; education is life itself."
John Dewey

Why Discharge Instructions are Important

Discharge instructions teach patients how to care for themselves and how to prevent complications after discharge from the hospital and outpatient procedures. Discharge instructions are necessary because when most patients are discharged from the hospital, they are not completely healed and may not be out of the danger zone.

Twenty percent of patients surveyed for a 2003 Annals of Medicine study said they became worse after discharge from the hospital and needed emergency care. The problems resulted in more pain and suffering, increased costs, permanent disability, and even death. The study went on to reveal some of the pain and suffering the patients experienced could have been avoided with proper discharge instructions. Discharge instructions are a very important part of your total care plan.

From what I have seen as a professional nurse, a caregiver, and a patient, I do not believe patients or providers fully appreciate the importance of discharge instructions. It has been my experience that nurses wait until just before the patient is about to be wheeled to the door and family members are in and out of the room carrying bags and making last minute room checks ("Hey, Ma, did you get your notebook out of the drawer? You got your prescriptions?) to give the discharge instructions. This is not an optimal time for learning. To be as safe as you can be after discharge, you need good discharge instructions. These instructions should be given the attention they warrant because they could help protect your health and safety.

How to Get Really Good Discharge Instructions

Your role as team leader:

- **Take your discharge instructions seriously.** Do not dismiss your discharge instructions as a last minute annoyance.

- **Ask well in advance of discharge for equipment instructions.** If you are going to go home with equipment or new appliances, your nurses or nurse educators will need to teach you how to care for yourself and your equipment at home. This training should happen days in advance of your discharge so you and your caregivers have time to ask questions and to get answers about how to care for you. You will want to practice what you will have to do at home while you have the nurses' support and your nurse is able to ensure you that you are performing procedures in the best way possible.

- **Ask for a specialist.** Many hospitals employ nurse specialists in the areas of diabetes, ostomy and wound care, and stroke to name a few. Nursing educators have advanced knowledge in their specialty areas and are excellent teachers. Ask for a nurse specialist to train you in caring for any equipment or devices you may have.

Questions to Help You Get Really Good Discharge Instructions

- **What happened to me and what did the team do to or for me while I was in the hospital?**

If you had surgery, the discharge instructions should include the name of the surgery and a brief synopsis of what was done during the surgery. If you had an infection, the type of antibiotics and other care you received for that infection should be described in your discharge instructions. You need this information to complete your history and update your PHR. It is your responsibility as the leader of **YOUR** Healthcare Team to know what happened to you.

- **What are my medications? Was I started on any new medications?**

Obtain written information about any new prescriptions including how to take them; when to take them; when not to take them; how long to take them; side effects; and the telephone number of the person who wrote the prescription so that you can call him if you have a problem. If your prescriptions have been emailed to the pharmacy, remember to get a printout of your prescriptions to compare with what the pharmacist gives you. (Remember to use your pharmacy and medication error prevention questions whenever you are given a new prescription.)

- **How do I care for my equipment?**

You may be discharged from the hospital with drains, tubes, dressings, collection bags, or any number of things you will care for at home that you did not have before your hospital stay. Be sure that you receive written instructions, whenever possible, that explain how to care for your new accessories and what do in the event the equipment malfunctions.

- **What are my activity instructions?**

Your discharge instructions should include when you can get out of bed, lift, take a shower, get in the tub, climb stairs, have sex, drive, and go back to work.

- **What are my dietary instructions?**

These instructions should include what you should and should not eat. If you are currently restricted from certain foods, ask when, if ever you can eat those foods again.

- **How will I know if I have a problem?**

The most commonly sited signs and symptoms of a problem are fever, pain, and swelling, all of which are signs and symptoms of an infection. You should also be taught the signs and symptoms of problems specific to your condition. For example, if you were admitted to the hospital with a breathing problem, you will want to know the breathing patterns that indicate you have a problem at home, and what you should do if that situation arises and you should be given a number to call in case a problem does arise.

- **When will I go to see my doctor?**

You should be told when you to see each of your doctors. In two days? One week? Or is no follow-up required? Whatever the time frame, it should be put in writing on your discharge instructions.

- **Will I need to follow up with any testing?**

You should be given a list of any pending tests and how to get the results of those tests. You should also be told if you need to schedule any tests or procedures after discharge and why you need those tests.

- **Will I be receiving home care?**

This information should include what, if any, homecare services you will need: nursing, physical therapy, nursing attendants, home blood work, IV maintenance, etc. The instructions should include how to get in touch with the service provider, when to expect the service, and how long you will receive the service.

- **May I have a copy of the discharge instructions?**

A copy of your discharge instructions will be put into your chart and made a part of your legal medical record. If you have a problem that results in injury after discharge, the hospital will produce a copy of your discharge instructions to prove you were given the information you needed to care for yourself safely at home. If you were not given proper discharge instructions, you on the other hand can say "They never told me that." The hospital, then, may be responsible for any damages that occur because you were not given proper discharge instructions; therefore it is important that you keep a signed copy of your discharge instructions in your PHR.

IN CONCLUSION

There are so many problems in healthcare: poor doctor patient communication, flawed record keeping, lack of time, lack of knowledge on behalf of patients, and unsafe practitioners are only some of the problems that plague our healthcare system and the dangers are lurking everywhere. Each of us is at risk of being hurt or harmed by a medical error everytime we enter the healthcare system no matter which door we enter through.

While the leaders in healthcare are documenting the numbers and debating the best ways to develop a culture of safety inside our healthcare system patients are dying by the hundreds of thousands, with no end in sight, the truth be told the numbers are getting worse.

It is my hope that after reading this book you will be able to prevent a medical error from happening to you and your loved ones by embracing your role as leader of *YOUR* Healthcare Team. I hope this book will help you to communicate more effectively with your doctors and to get the correct diagnosis and the best treatments possible. Treatment you participated in choosing; treatment that meets all of your unique needs; and treatment with which you can be satisfied. I hope this book helps you to be safe and free from all the suffering our healthcare system has to offer.

APPENDIX

Worksheets

The worksheets in this section can be copied as many times as you like and taken with you to all of the appointments. To help you understand why you need answers to the following questions, refer to the chapter from which the worksheet originated and review the rationale given for asking each question. Once the worksheets are completed, you can review them with your doctors and family members and keep them for your own information. You may even want to make the answers part of your PHR.

O.L.D.C.A.R.T.S Practice Sheet

Use this form to describe and document the symptoms associated with your current ailment. After you have documented your symptoms, practice telling your story in a clear and concise manner using the information recorded on this worksheet as a guide.

Onset: When did your symptoms first begin? How did they start? Was it after you ate? Did you hurt yourself? Were you "stressed out?"

_____

_____

Location of the problem: Where is the problem? To avoid confusion always point to the area of your body that is hurting and to the other parts of your body that are affected by your problem.

_____

_____

Duration: Duration includes two dimensions: how long do the symptoms last once they start (one hour, all day, they never stop) and how long has the condition itself been going on (one week, two months one year)? Think about and answer both parts of the question.

_____

_____

Characteristics: Is your pain colicky (does it come and go, produce gas, burping, or flatulence)? Is the pain, dull or sharp? Is it hot or stabbing?

_____

_____

Associated Symptoms: What other symptoms are associated with your problem? For example if you have a stomachache do you also have fever, chills, nausea, vomiting, diarrhea. Think about and then document the other symptoms associated with your chief complaint.

_____

_____

Relieving Factors/ Treatments Tried: What brings relief of your symptoms? Do your symptoms improve when you move, eat, drink tea, or take medication? Let the provider know what treatments you have tried, how they worked and how much relief you did or did not get from them.

_____

_____

Timing: Timing includes the actual time your symptoms occur and the relationship of your symptoms to other things. Do your symptoms start in the morning when you first get up or at night? Do they start after dinner or exercise? What is the timing of your symptoms?

_____

_____

Severity: Severity relates to pain and how the symptoms have affected your life and your ability to care for yourself. How bad is the pain on a scale of 1-10? Is it the worst pain you've ever experienced (a 10 or greater) or is the pain minor (a 2-3 on the pain scale)? How have your symptoms affected your life? Are you able to care for yourself? What abilities are you losing? Can you move without assistance, can you work? Are you able to perform your daily activities?

_____

_____

Whenever you are going to talk with a member of *YOUR* Healthcare Team put your symptoms into the O.L.D.C.A.R.T.S format and practice, practice, practice your presentation before the visit.

Questions to Ask When Choosing a Doctor

Many of these questions can be answered by the office staff or by researching the provider on the Internet (see Chapter Four for Website suggestions)

Is the provider part of your insurance plan?

Doctor A:_____

Doctor B:_____

Doctor C:_____

Is there a long wait to get an appointment?

Doctor A:_____

Doctor B:_____

Doctor C:_____

How long is the wait in the waiting room to see the doctor?

Doctor A:_____

Doctor B:_____

Doctor C:_____

How much time is scheduled for appointments?

Doctor A:_____

Doctor B:_____

Doctor C:_____

Does the clinician have the background and training you need? If you have a heart condition you may need a cardiologist: if you have a stomach problem you may need a gastroenterologist. Does the provider have the background and training you need?

Doctor A:_____

Doctor B:_____

Doctor C:_____

Is the provider board certified? Having board certification means the provider completed extra hours of clinical training and then completed an exam in his or her area of specialty in order to become board certified.

Doctor A:_____

Doctor B:_____

Doctor C:_____

Which hospital(s) does the doctor use? Are they hospitals to which you want to go? Are they covered by your plan?

Doctor A:_____

Doctor B:_____

Doctor C:_____

Does the provider take care of hospitalized patients? Or are his patients treated by a hospitalist (a provider on staff at the hospital who takes care of patients who do not have doctors or whose doctors do not come to the hospital to care for patients)?

Doctor A:_____

Doctor B:_____

Doctor C:_____

What are the provider's office hours? Having evening hours is important if you or your advocate work during the day.

Doctor A:_____

Doctor B:_____

Doctor C:_____

Does the doctor or someone else (whose job it is to translate) speak the language I am most comfortable speaking?

Doctor A:_____

Doctor B:_____

Doctor C:_____

Is the provider part of your native culture? Is this important to you?

Doctor A:_____

Doctor B:_____

Doctor C:_____

Who takes care of the doctors patients' when she is not available? Does that person have the training needed for my special condition(s)?

Doctor A:_____

Doctor B:_____

Doctor C:_____

Does the doctor take phone calls from patients or give advice over the phone if you can't make it to the office? If not can you always make it in to the office?

Doctor A:_____

Doctor B:_____

Doctor C:_____

Will the staff automatically call in refills or do you have to come in to pick up you new prescriptions? Can you afford the co-pay associated with those office visits?

Doctor A:_____

Doctor B:_____

Doctor C:_____

Is the provider male or female? Does that matter to you?

Doctor A:_____

Doctor B:_____

Doctor C:_____

What are the providers' religious views, do they matter to you? This could come into play in issues of women's health, birth control, and alternative methods of contraception.

Doctor A:_____

Doctor B:_____

Doctor C:_____

Does the doctors' age matter to you? (Which doctor is the age you prefer)?

Doctor A:_____

Doctor B:_____

Doctor C:_____

Questions to Ask Yourself After You Meet the Provider

You will only be able to answers these questions after a visit to the doctor. The answers to these questions reflect what you thought, felt, and experienced during the interview process. The answers will help you rate the doctors beside manner and to decide if the doctor is a good fit for you and what you want from a doctor.

Do you feel confident the doctor is safe and knowledgeable in the areas of care you need?

Doctor A:_____

Doctor B:_____

Doctor C:_____

Did the doctor listen to you and give you enough time to explain your problem without interrupting?

Doctor A:_____

Doctor B:_____

Doctor C:_____

Was it easy to talk to the doctor? Could you ask and answer questions easily? Did you feel comfortable talking to and with the doctor?

Doctor A:_____

Doctor B:_____

Doctor C:_____

Did the doctor respect your thoughts and opinions about your condition and encourage you to participate in the conversation about your care?

Doctor A:_____

Doctor B:_____

Doctor C:_____

Did the doctor answer your questions in terms you understood? Did she ask you questions to make sure you understood her explanations?

Doctor A:_____

Doctor B:_____

Doctor C:_____

s the provider a good teacher? Did she teach you about diet, exercise, rest, and therapy, or did she just discuss medications?

    Doctor A:_____

    Doctor B:_____

    Doctor C:_____

Did she ask you your preferences about different kinds of treatments and seem open to your ideas? Did she explain the pros and cons of your choices?

    Doctor A:_____

    Doctor B:_____

    Doctor C:_____

Did the doctor spend enough time with you and give you his or her undivided attention?

    Doctor A:_____

    Doctor B:_____

    Doctor C:_____

Did you see the doctor wash his or her hands between examining patients?

    Doctor A:_____

    Doctor B:_____

    Doctor C:_____

Questions to Help You Understand Your Diagnosis and Treatment Options

What is my diagnosis, its medical name, and what it means in plain English?

_____

_____

Is additional testing needed before you are sure of the diagnosis or are you sure now?

_____

_____

What are my treatment options?

_____

_____

What are the benefits of each of my treatment options?

_____

_____

What are the risks associated with each of my treatment options?

_____

_____

Which option do you recommend considering my age, gender, culture, and my ability to tolerate the treatment?

_____

_____

In what percentage of cases is each of my options successful?

_____

_____

What do you consider successful?

_____

_____

Have you treated patients in the way you are suggesting? How are those patients doing now?

_____

_____

How long does it take to get results from each of the treatment options?

_____

_____

How many treatments will I need?

_____

_____

Is the treatment you suggest covered by my insurance?

_____

_____

What happens if I choose to have no treatment at all?

_____

_____

How will we manage the side effects of my treatment?

_____

_____

Will I have pain? If so, how will you manage it?

_____

_____

Am I contagious? If so, what should those affected do?

_____

_____

Is my condition genetic? If so, what should my family members know about this condition?

_____

_____

Should I see a specialist?

_____

_____

Who do you recommend?

_____

_____

How will this affect my life?

_____

_____

Will I need education, counseling, nursing care, family support, physical therapy, or any other type of help to cope with my illness?

_____

_____

Is there anything I should do to monitor myself? Should I take my blood pressure, monitor my blood sugar, check my weight, count my calories, or have routine laboratory work?

_____

_____

What are the normal results of the testing? When should I call you with an abnormal result?

_____

_____

Is there anyone who can teach me to do the monitoring?

_____

_____

In your opinion what will happen to me during this illness?

_____

_____

Will I be able to work?

_____

_____

How long will I need to be out of work?

_____

_____

Can you help me complete my disability forms?

_____

_____

Do you recommend any natural therapies like massage, aromatherapy, vitamins, supplements, yoga, acupuncture, meditation, change in diet, ect.? How will they help me?

_____

_____

Are there any educational or support groups to help me learn more about and cope with my condition?

_____

_____

Questions to Help You Decide Between Two or More Treatment Options

Do you think you can you tolerate the treatment and its side effects? Do you want to tolerate the treatments long and short-term side effects?

_____

_____

What will your recovery entail? Will you need nursing care? Will you need to go to a rehabilitation facility? Will you need someone to drive you around and shop for you?

_____

_____

Do you have the support needed for your care? Will your insurance carrier help you find the care and services you need? Can family members or friends help you?

_____

_____

How far is the treatment from your home?

_____

_____

Can you travel to the treatment location by yourself?

_____

_____

For each of the possible options ask yourself, "What if the worst thing that can happen does happen, can I live with that?"

_____

_____

Eliminate the options with side effects or outcomes you find unacceptable and you do not want to live with.

_____

_____

Questions to Help Prevent Medication and Pharmacy Errors

What is the name of the medicine and how do you spell it?

_____

_____

Why am I taking the drug? (high blood pressure, diabetes, blood thinning)

_____

_____

What dose are you prescribing? If at all possible can you write the prescription without using decimal points.

_____

_____

How many times per day should I take the medicine and how many hours apart should I take the doses? Does twice a day mean every twelve hours or at 10.a.m. and 6 p.m.?

_____

_____

What are the side effects of the drug? Ask the pharmacist to evaluate your medications for interactions with your other medications.

_____

_____

What side effects will tell me I should stop taking the medication and call you to let you know about them?

_____

_____

How long do I need to take the medicine?

_____

_____

When will the medication start working?

_____

_____

Can I stop taking my medicine if I feel better?

_____

_____

Should I avoid any food, drinks, or activities while on the medication?

_____

_____

Should the medicine be taken with food or on an empty stomach?

_____

_____

Is there anything I need to monitor at home: blood pressure, blood sugar, urine output, mood, heart rate, or anything else? If so what are the normal levels of each measurement and at what levels should I call you?

_____

_____

When should I have lab work done and how often should it be repeated?

_____

_____

Can I take a generic version of this medication? A generic is a non-brand name, less expensive version of the drug.

_____

_____

Questions to Ask When Laboratory Tests are Ordered

What are the test(s) for and why do we need the results?

_____

_____

What will the results tell us? Too much iron, too little hemoglobin, too much salt? How will the results contribute to my care?

_____

_____

How should I prepare for the test? Do you have written instructions?

_____

_____

Who will perform the test? How much experience does he or she have performing this procedure?

_____

_____

Is the test painful? If it is not customary to give pain medication and you know you are not the best with handling pain, ask for special consideration and ask to be given pain medication in advance of the treatment.

_____

_____

Should the test be done at a specialty lab?

_____

_____

How often will the test need to be repeated? Every six months? Once per year? How often?

_____

_____

When will we get the results? If you are not called or notified of the test results when you anticipated, call the provider who performed the test and request your test results.

_____

_____

Can we recheck the results to make sure they are accurate? If your lab results are vastly different from previous lab test results, ask for another set of labs to be drawn to see which set rendered an accurate result.

_____

_____

What are the next steps after we get the test results?

_____

_____

Questions to Help You Choose the Best Hospital

Does the hospital specialize in treating my condition? How well do their patients do compared with other hospitals in my area?

_____

_____

How does the hospital compare with others in my area?

_____

_____

Is this hospital covered by my health insurance? If the hospital is not covered by your plan and you need specialized care that can only be given at the specialty hospital, call your insurance carrier and ask to speak to the case manager or patient advocate. Ask if she can negotiate a contract with the hospital for your care.

_____

_____

Does my doctor have privileges (is he or she allowed to work) at the hospital of my choice? If you are not going to have your regular doctor at a specialty hospital, this may be a trade-off for seeing an expert who specializes in your care.

Questions to Help You Choose the Best Surgeon and Hospital for Your Surgery

Is the surgeon board certified in the type of surgery you are having?

_____

_____

How much experience does the surgeon have performing this type of operation? What is the surgeons' success rate in this area of surgery? Who will assist him in the surgery and how well qualified is each assistant?

_____

_____

At which hospital will the operation be done? How often is the same operation performed there? Research shows that patients do better when they have surgery in hospitals that specialize in the type of surgery and post-operative care they need.

_____

_____

Questions to Help You Get Fully Informed Surgical Consent

Why do I need surgery?

_____

_____

What kind of surgery do I need?

_____

_____

What will you be doing while you are inside me? How will you rearrange my parts?

_____

_____

What are the benefits and risks of having this surgery?

_____

_____

How successful is this surgery?

_____

_____

What do you consider successful?

_____

_____

Is there some other way to treat my condition or is there another surgical procedure I can choose? What are the risks and benefits of that option?

_____

_____

How will the surgery make my life better and for how long?

_____

_____

How will the surgery make my life worse and for how long?

_____

_____

How much pain will I have after the surgery and how do you or the pain management team plan to control my pain?

_____

_____

Will I need general anesthesia? Can I have something else? If you can have regional or local anesthesia it could be a safer choice. Safety is always first.

_____

_____

How long will the surgery take? This speaks to how much time you will spend under anesthesia and how much risk you face.

_____

_____

Will I wake up with any tubes, drains, or special equipment attached to me?

_____

_____

How long will I have this equipment?

_____

_____

Will it be necessary for someone teach to me how to care for my tube, drains, bandages, etc?.

_____

_____

How long will it take me to recover? Will I need rehabilitation or nursing care at home?

_____

_____

How long will I be in the hospital?

_____

_____

How much will the surgery cost?

_____

_____

Will my health insurance cover the costs of the surgery?

_____

_____

What will happen if I wait or if I choose not to have this surgery?

_____

_____

Where can I get a second opinion? Getting a second opinion is highly recommended before any surgery.

_____

_____

Questions to Help You Get Really Good Discharge Instructions

What happened while I was in the hospital?

_____

_____

Who can teach me how to care for myself and my new equipment at home?

_____

_____

Do you have written information about my care that I can take home with me?

_____

_____

What are my medications? How do I take them and at what time? When should I not take them? What are the side effects?

_____

_____

Was I started on any new medications? Am I being discharged on those new medications? Do you have my prescriptions? If they have been emailed to the pharmacy remember to get a printout of them to compare with what the pharmacist gave you and remember to use your medication error prevention questions whenever you are given new medications.

_____

_____

What are my activity instructions? When can I shower? When can I go up and down stairs? When can I go back to work? When can I have sex? When can I drive?

_____

_____

What are my diet instructions? Is there anything I shouldn't eat? When will the food restrictions be lifted. What should I be eating?

_____

_____

How do I know if I have a problem? What would be the signs and symptoms? When do I call for help?

_____

_____

Am I waiting for the results of any outstanding tests?

_____

_____

Am I scheduled for any follow up testing?

_____

_____

When am I scheduled to see my doctor(s)?

_____

_____

Who do I call for help? (Be sure you have the name and number of that person).

_____

_____

Depression Assessment

Depression Assessment	Yes	No
Do you have feelings of: sadness, isolation, hopelessness, or guilt most of the time? Are people complaining that you are irritable or cranky?		
Do you feel isolated and alone even when people are around?		
Have you lost interest in things that used to bring you joy like hobbies, relationships, sex, or work?		
Are you sleeping too much or too little? Are you tired most of the time?		
Are you having trouble managing your high blood pressure, diabetes, or stomach ailments?		

Do you have unexplained muscle or joint pain, backaches, or headaches?		
Are you eating too much or too little? Do you have a sudden weight gain or loss?		
Are you having thoughts of **suicide?** If so, call your doctor or go to the emergency room and **GET HELP IMMEDIATELY.**		

Provider Visit Flow Sheet

Date and Time of Visit	Name of Provider	Comments About Exam	Test Results	Next Steps (Labs, tests, therapy...)

REFERENCES

AARP. Medical error and patient injury: Costly and often preventable. Retrieved January 11, 2009 from http://www. aarp.org/research/health/carequality/Articles/aresearch-import-711-IB35.html - DRUGS

About.com. Advanced care directives. Retrieved April 26, 2009 from http://adam.about.com/encyclopedia/Advanced-care-directives.htm

About.com. Depression symptoms. Retrieved April 15, 2009 from http://depression.about.com/od/diagnosis/Depression_Symptoms.htm

About.com. Effective patient-doctor communication. Retrieved January 10, 2009 from http://patients.about.com/od/therightdoctorforyou/a/docpatientcomm.htm

About.com. Health topics A-Z: Advanced care directives. Retrieved January 11, 2009 from http://adam.about.com/encyclopedia/Advanced-care-directives.htm

About.com. How to choose the right doctor for you. Retrieved January 11, 2009 from http://arthritis.about.com/cs/docpad/ht/choosedoctor.htm

About.com. How would you rate your doctor? Retrieved January 11, 2009 from http://arthritis.about.com/cs/docpad/a/rateyourdoctor.htm

About.com. MRSA and other super bug infections. Retrieved January 11, 2009 from http://patients.about.com/od/atthehospital/a/hais.htm

About.com. Review your medical records for errors: Fixing these mistakes can have an impact on your diagnosis and treatment. Retrieved April 14, 2009 from http://patients.about.com/od/yourmedicalrecords/a/correcterrors.htm

About.com. Should You Change Doctors? "C" if your needs are being met. Retrieved January 10, 2009 from http://arthritis.about.com/cs/docpad/a/changedoc.htm

About.com. The patient-physician encounter. Retrieved January 11, 2009 from http://arthritis.about.com/cs/docpad/a/patientdoctor.htm

About.com. Top 10 reasons to fire your doctor. Retrieved January 11, 2009 from

http://arthritis.about.com/od/buildyourhealthcareteam/tp/fireyourdoctor.htm

About.com. Understanding informed consent: Be sure you understand before you sign on the dotted line. Retrieved January 11, 2009 from http://patients.about.com/od/yourmedicalrecords/a/informedconsent.htm

About.com. Using health website symptom checkers. Retrieved January 11, 2009 from http://patients.about.com/od/yourdiagnosis/a/symptomcheck.htm

Administrators In Medicine. Docfinder searches. Retrieved January 11, 2009 from http://www.docboard.org

Advocate Health Care. Advocate doctor directory. Retrieved January 10, 2009 from http://www.advocatehealth.com/db/physref/

Agency for Healthcare Research and Quality. Be prepared for medical appointments. Retrieved April 21, 2009 from http://www.ahrq.gov/qual/beprepared.pdf

Agency for Healthcare Research and Quality. Choosing a doctor. Retrieved January 11, 2009 from http://www.ahcpr. gov/consumer/qntascii/qntdr.htm-decide%23decide

Agency for Healthcare Research and Quality. Choosing a hospital. Retrieved January 10, 2009 from http://www.ahrq. gov/consumer/qnt/qnthosp.htm - choosing

Agency for Healthcare Research and Quality. Consumers and Patients. Retreived April 13, 2009 from http://www.ahrq.gov/ consumer/

Agency for Healthcare Research and Quality. Diagnosing diagnosis errors: Lessons from a multi-institutional collaborative project. Retreived January 11, 2009 from http:// www.ahrq.gov/downloads/pub/advances/vol2/Schiff.pdf

Agency for Healthcare Research and Quality. Efforts to reduce medical errors: AHRQ's response to senate committee on appropriations questions. Retrieved January 11, 2009 from http://www.ahrq.gov/qual/pscongrpt/psini2. htm#HowRecord

Agency for Healthcare Research and Quality. Making sure your surgery is safe. Retreived January 11, 2009 from http:// www.ahrq.gov/consumer/surgery/surgery6.htm

Agency for Healthcare Research and Quality. Many errors by medical residents caused by teamwork breakdowns, lack of supervision. Retrieved April 21, 2009 from

http://www.ahrq.gov/news/press/pr2007/teambreakpr.htm

Agency for Healthcare Research and Quality.Medical errors and patient safety. Retreived January 11, 2009 from http://www.ahrq.gov/qual/errorsix.htm - docs

Agency for Healthcare Research and Quality. Making sure your surgery is safe. Retreived April 26, 2009 from http://www.ahrq.gov/consumer/surgery/surgery6.htm

Agency for Healthcare Research and Quality. Medical errors, the scope of the problem: An epidemic of errors. Retreived January 11, 2009 from http://www.ahrq.gov/qual/errback.htm

Agency for Healthcare Research and Quality. Questions are the answers: Get more involved with your healthcare. Retreived January 10, 2009 from http://www.ahrq.gov/questionsaretheanswer

Agency for Healthcare Research and Quality. Quick tips – when talking with your doctor. Retreived January 11, 2009 from http://www.ahrq.gov/consumer/quicktips/doctalk.htm

Agency for Healthcare Research and Quality. 20 Tips To Help Prevent Medical Errors. Retrieved January 11, 2009 from http://www.ahrq.gov/consumer/20tips.htm

Agency for Healthcare Research and Quality. Patients safety network.glossary. Retrieved April 14, 2009 from http://psnet. ahrq.gov/glossary.aspx#F

American Bar Association. Health Care Advance Directives. Retrieved April 26, 2009 from http://www.abanet.org/ publiced/practical/directive_planning.htm

American Cancer Society. Informed consent. Retrieved January 11, 2009 from http://www.cancer.org/docroot/ETO/ content/ETO_1_2X_Informed_Consent.asp

American College of Surgeons. Public information. Retreived April 21, 2009 from http://www.facs.org/public_info/ppserv. html

American Medical Association. Retreived January 11, 2009 from http://www.amaassn.org/

Answers.com. Preventable medical errors. Retrieved January 10, 2009 from http://www.answers.com/topic/preventable-medical-errors

AOLHealth.com. Sticking with treatment-overcoming barriers to treatment: Depression. Retrieved April 16, 2009 from http://www.aolhealth.com/depression/learn-aboutit/overcoming-barriers-to-treatment/sticking-with-treatment

Be Med Wise: Being med wise helps us use medications safely. Retrieved January 10, 2009 from http://www.bemedwise.org/

Besen, Aaron. 2008. Hospitals to loose never event reimbursement." *VBJ Online,* April 4. Retrieved Janary 13, 2009 from http://www.vbjusa.com/stories/2008-0404/hospitals_to_lose_never_event_reimbursement.html

Beyea, S.C. 2007. Distractions, interruptions, and patient safety. *AORN,* 86: 109-110,112.

Blanton-Lillie, M., Rushing, O.E. & Ruiz, S. (2003). Key facts, race, ethnicity & medical care. The Henry J. Kaiser Family Foundation. Retrieved April 16, 2009 from http://www.kff.org/minorityhealth/upload/Key-Facts-Race-Ethnicity-Medical-Care-Chartbook.pdf

Centers For Medical Consumers. Hospital-acquired infections-protect yourself. http://www.medicalconsumers.org/pages/Hospital-acquiredinfections.html (accessed January 10, 2009).

Centers for Medicare and Medicaid Services. Eliminating serious, preventable, and costly medical errors – never events.

http://www.cms.hhs.gov/apps/media/press/release. asp?Counter=1863

Centers for Medicare and Medicaid Services. Getting a second opinion before surgery. http://www.medicare.gov/ publications/pubs/pdf/02173.pdf (accessed January 11, 2009).

Clarke, J.R., Johnston, E. Finley, J. 2007. Getting surgery right. *Annals of Surgery* 246: 395-405.

Cluett, J. 2007. Pre-operative questions. Retreived April 25, 2009 from http://orthopedics.about.com/cs/ jointreplacement1/a/questions.htm

Combes, Alain, et al. 2004. Clinical and autopsy diagnoses in the intensive care unit a prospective study. *Archives of Intern Medicine.*164: 389-392.

CureResearch.com. Causes of medical mistakes. Retreived January 11, 2009 from http://www.cureresearch.com/ mistakes/causes.htm

Cure Research. Over-diagnosed diseases. http://www. cureresearch.com/intro/overdiag.htm (accessed January 11, 2009).

CVS Caremark. Ill's and conditions special report: Avoiding pharmacy errors. http://healthresources.caremark.com/topic/ rxtrouble (accessed January 11, 2009).

Davenport, J. 2000. Documenting high-risk cases to avoid malpractice liability. *Family Practice Management* (October).

Delbanco, T. & Bell, S.K. 2007. Guilty, afraid, and alone – struggling with medical error. *New England Journal of Medicine* 357: 1682-1683. http://content.nejm.org.libproxy2. umdnj.edu/cgi/content/full/357/17/1682

Department of Veterans Affairs Health Services Research & Development Service: Evidence synthesis pilot program. Racial and ethnic disparities in the VA healthcare system: A systematic review. http://www.hsrd.research.va.gov/ publications/esp/RacialDisparities2007.pdf (accessed April 1, 2009).

Diagnose Me.com. The analyst. http://www.diagnose-me. com (accessed January 11, 2009).

diagKNOWsis. Working with medical and other professionals. http://www.diagknowsis.org/professionals.htm (accessed April 2, 2009).

Do Your Proxy.org. Create your advance directive documents online, for free. http://www.doyourproxy.com (accessed April 2, 2009).

Douglas, R.S. 2009. The direct medical costs of healthcare-associated infections in U.S. hospitals and the benefits of prevention http://patients.about.com/gi/dynamic/offsite.htm?zi=1/XJ&sdn=patients&cdn=health&tm=11&f=22&su=p284.9.336.ip_p736.8.336.ip_&tt=2&bt=0&bts=1&zu=http%3A//www.cdc.gov/ncidod/dhqp/hai.html

Drug Information Online Drugs.com http://www.drugs.com (accessed January 11, 2009).

Ducel, G, et., al 2002. Prevention of hospital-acquired infections: A practical guide. World Health Organization http://www.who.int/csr/resources/publications/whocdscsreph200212.pdf

Elliot, R.L. 2007. Depression in primary care. *Ethnicity and Disease* 17:28-33

Encyclopedia of Surgery: A guide for patients and caregivers. Discharge from the hospital. http://www.surgeryencyclopedia.

com/Ce-Fi/Discharge-from-the-hospital.html (accessed January 11, 2009).

Foreman, J. 2006. For when doctors and a nurse just aren't enough. Boston Globe, May 2006 http://www.boston.com/news/globe/health_science/articles/2006/05/01/for_when_a_doctor_and_a_nurse_just_arent_enough/?page=2 (no longer accessible)

Forster, A. J., et al. 2003. The incidence and severity of adverse events affecting patients after discharge from the hospital. *Annals of Internal Medicine,* 138: 161–167.

Fortinberry, A. The 3 essentials for building successful relationships. *Uplift Program.* http://www.upliftprogram.com/article_relatetip.html (accessed January 10, 2009)

Fuhrmans, V. 2008. Insurers stop paying for hospital errors. The Wall Street Journal. http://www.azcentral.com/business/consumer/articles/0115biz-insurersmistake15-ON.html

Golden, S.H. et al. 2004. Depressive symptoms and the risk of type 2 diabetes: The atherosclerosis risk in communities study. *Diabetes Care* 27: 429-435.

HealthGrades 2004. Patient safety in American hospitals http://www.healthgrades.com/media/english/pdf/HG_

Patient_Safety_Study_Final.pdf (accessed January 11, 2009).

HealthGrades. 2005 Medical-errors gap widens between best and worst hospitals: HealthGrades study. http://www.healthgrades.com/media/DMS/pdf/ DHAPSNationalReleaseFINAL4May022005.pdf

HealthGrades. 2006. HealthGrades quality study third annual patient safety in American hospitals study April 2006. http://www.healthgrades.com/media/dms/pdf/ PatientSafetyInAmericanHospitalsStudy2006.pdf

HealthGrades.com. Research physicians. http://www. Healthgrades.com (accessed January10, 2009).

HealthPages.com. http://www.thehealthpages.com (accessed January 10, 2009).

Hospital Buyer. Non-payment for never events gaining momentum with insurers. http://www.hospitalbuyer.com/ industry-market/non-payment-for-never-events-gaining- momentum-with-insurers-2145/ (accessed January 11, 2009).

iHealthBeat. 2007. Physicians tackle medical chart errors in online forum. http://www.ihealthbeat.org/articles/2007/11/26/

Physicians-Tackle-Medical-Chart-Errors-in-Online-Forum. aspx?topicID=53 (accessed April 26, 2009)

Institute for Safe Medication Practices. Medication Safety Alert! http://www.ismp.org/Newsletters/acutecare/articles/19990407.asp (accessed January 11, 2009)

Institute of Medicine. Health literacy: A prescription to end confusion. http://iom.edu/CMS/3775/3827/19723.aspx (accessed January 11, 2009).

Institute of Medicine. 2006. Preventing medication errors. http://www.iom.edu/Object.File/Master/35/943/medication%20errors%20new.pdf (accessed April 20, 2009)

Institute of Medicine 2006. What you can do to avoid medication errors. http://www.iom.edu/Object.File/Master/35/945/medication%20errors%20fact%20sheet.pdf (accessed January 11, 2009).

Institute of Medicine. 2002. To err is human: Building a safer health system. http://www.nap.edu/openbook. php?isbn=0309068371(accessed January 11, 2009).

The Institute for Safe Medication Practices 1999. The five rights. http://www.ismp.org/Newsletters/acutecare/articles/19990407.asp (accessed April 20, 2009

Johnson, Rachel, L. (2004). Patient race/ethnicity and quality of patient-physician communication during medical visits. American Journal of Public Health. http://www.ajph.org/cgi/content/abstract/94/12/2084(accessed April 19, 2009).

Joint Commission. Helping you choose the hospital for you. http://www.jointcommission.org/GeneralPublic/Choices/hc_hap.htm (accessed January 11, 2009).

Joint Commission. What did the doctor say: Improving health literacy to protect patient safety. http://www.jointcommission.org/NR/rdonlyres/F53D5057-5349-4391-9DB9-E7F086873D46/0/health_literacy_exec_summary.pdf (accessed January, 9, 2009)

Kaiser Family Foundation. Minority Health. http://www.kff.org/minorityhealth/index.cfm (accessed January 11, 2009).

Kozier, B., Erb, G., & Blais, K. *Concepts and Issues in Nursing Practice.* CA: Addison-Wesley Nursing.

Kronz, J.D., Westra, H. & Epstein, J.I. 1999. Mandatory second opinion surgical pathology at a large referral hospital. *Cancer.* 86: 2426-2435.

LawDepot.com. Health Care Directive. http:lawdepot.com (accessed April 26, 2009)

Lapid, M. & T. Rummans. 2003. "Evaluation and management of geriatric depression in primary care. *Mayo Clinical Proceedings* 78: 1423-1429.

Leap Frog Group. https://leapfrog.org (accessed January 13, 2009)

Leape, L.L. 1994. Error in medicine. *JAMA* 272: 1851-1857.

Levine, E. How to choose your doctor. http://www.enotalone. com/article/4994.html (accessed April 26, 2009)

Meyers, K. Issue Brief: Racial and ethnic health disparities. Institute for Health Policy. http://www.kpihp.org/publications/ docs/disparities_highlights.pdf (accessed April 16, 2009)

Murray, B. & Fortinberry, A. Depression facts and stats. *Uplift Program.* http://www.upliftprogram.com/depression_ stats.html#23 (accessed January 10, 2009).

Murray, B. Mind and body. *Uplift Program.* http://www. upliftprogram.com/h_mindbody_03.html#h30 (accessed April 15, 2009)

myPHR.com. Free health record forms. http://www.myphr. com/your_record/free_forms.asp (accessed January 11, 2009).

National Academies of Health Sciences. Medication errors injure 1.5 million people and cost billions of dollars annually. http://www8.nationalacademies.org/onpinews/newsitem.aspx?RecordID=11623 (accessed January 11, 2009).

National Conference of State Legislatures. "Never events" become ever present as more states refuse to pay for mistakes. http://www.ncsl.org/programs/health/shn/2008/sn519b.htm (accessed January 11, 2009).

National Coordinating Council for Medication Error Reporting and Prevention. About medication errors. http://www.nccmerp.org/aboutMedErrors.html (accessed January 10, 2009).

National Guideline Clearinghouse. http://www.guideline.gov (accessed January 11, 2009).

National Institute of Mental Health. Depression: A treatable illness. http://www.nimh.nih.gov/health/publications/depression-a-treatable-illness.shtml (accessed January 10, 2009).

National Network of Libraries of Medicine. Health Literacy. http://nnlm.gov/outreach/consumer/hlthlit.html (accessed January 11, 2009).

National Patient Safety Foundation at the AMA. Public opinion of patient safety issues research findings. http://www.npsf.org/download/1997survey.pdf (accessed January 11, 2009).

O'Rielly, K.B. 2008. No pay for "never event" errors becoming standard. Amednews.com: American Medical News. http://www.ama-assn.org/amednews/2008/01/07/prsc0107.htm (accessed April 26, 2009)

Physician Reports. http://www.physicianreports.com. (accessed April 25, 2009)

RateMDs.com. Give your doctor a checkup. http://www.ratemds.com/social/ (accessed January 11, 2009).

RID Committee To Reduce Infection Deaths. 15 steps you can take to reduce your risk of a hospital infection.http://www.hospitalinfection.org/protectyourself.shtml (accessed January 11, 2009).

Robert Wood Johnson Foundation. Patient illiteracy affects compliance with healthcare instructions.http://www.rwjf.org/reports/grr/030763s.htm (accessed January 11, 2009).

Roizen, M.R. & Oz, M.C. 2006. *You: The Smart Patient.* New York: Free Press.

Science Daily. Doctors under-reporting medical errors to hospitals.(2008)___ http://www.sciencedaily.com/releases/2008/01/080114162532.htm (accessed January 11, 2009).

Science Daily. Study highlights the ramifications of medical misdiagnosis. http://www.sciencedaily.com/releases/2005/11/051107075616.htm (accessed April 26, 2009

Seattlepi.com. Doctors order needless tests say experts. http://seattlepi.nwsource.com/health/270925_needlesstests20.html (accessed January 11, 2009).

Smedley, B.D et al. (2003). Unequal Treatment. Confronting racial and ethnic disparities in health care, executive summary. http://www.allhealth.org/BriefingMaterials/UnequalTreatment-56.pdf

Stoppler, M. & Hecht, B. How to choose a doctor. http://www.medicinenet.com/script/main/art.asp?articlekey=4764 accessed April 25, 2009)

St. Peter's University Hospital. How to Choose A Doctor http://www.medicinenet.com/script/main/art.asp?articlekey=47649 (accessed January 11, 2008)

Torrey, T. 2008. Are you seeing the right specialist? http://patients.about.com/od/misdiagnosis/a/rightspecialist.htm (accessed April 26, 2009)

Torrey, T. 2007. Differential Diagnosis: What else might your illness be? http://patients.about.com/od/yourdiagnosis/a/diffdiagnosis.htm (accessed April 26, 2009)

Torrey, T. 2008. Medical treatment decision making: Taking responsibility. http://patients.about.com/od/researchtreatmentoptions/a/decisionmaking.htm. (accessed April 21,2009)

Torrey, T. 2008. MRSA and other superbug infections. http://patients.about.com/od/atthehospital/a/hais.htm

Torrey, T. 2007. Using health website symptom checkers. http://patients.about.com/od/yourdiagnosis/a/symptomcheck.htm

Torrey, T. 2008. Misdiagnois—What is Misdiagnosis? http://patients.about.com/od/misdiagnosis/a/defmisdiagnosis.htm (accessed April 26, 2009)

Torrey, T. 2008. Your role as a partner on your healthcare team. http://patients.about.com/od/researchtreatmentoptions/a/hcteam.htm (April 26, 2009)

Torrey, T. 2008. What is a medical error. http://patients.about.com/od/atthehospital/a/mederrorlist.htm (access April 26, 2009)

Torrey, T. 2008. Why don't patients comply with treatment recommendations? http://patients.about.com/od/decisionmaking/a/noncompliance.htm (accessed April 20, 2008

U Compare Health Care. Find a doctor. http://www.ucomparehealthcare.com/physicians_start.html (accessed January 10, 2009).

United States Department of Health and Human Services. Health literacy and health outcomes. http://www.health.gov/communication/literacy/quickguide/factsliteracy.htm - eighteen (accessed January 10, 2009)

United States Department of Health and Human Services. Healthfinder.gov. http://www.healthfinder.gov (accessed January 11, 2009).

United States Food and Drug Administration. Make no mistake: Medical errors can be deadly serious. http://www.fda.gov/fdac/features/2000/500_err.html (accessed January11, 2009).

WebMd. Healthcare agents: Appointing one and being one."
http://www.webmd.com/a-to-z-guides/health-care-agents-
appointing-one-being-one (accessed January 10, 2009).

University of Iowa Hospitals and Clinics (2008). Medical
Error Disconnect. http://www.uihealthcare.com/news/
pacemaker/2008/spring/medicalerrors.html (accessed January
15, 2009)

WebMd. Healthcare Agents: Appointing one and being one.
http://www.webmd.com/a-to-z-guides/health-care-agents-
appointing-one-being-one (accessed April 26, 2009).

WebMd. The living will and durable power of attorney for
healthcare. http://www.webmd.com/a-to-z-guides/frequently-
asked-questions-about-advanced-directives (accessed January
11, 2009).

WebMd. Questions and answers about depression. http://
www.webmd.com/depression/questions-and-answers-about-
depression (accessed January 11, 2009).

Williams, E.S. et al., 2007. The relationship of organizational
culture, stress, satisfaction, and burnout with physician-
reported error and suboptimal patient care: Results from the
MEMO study. *Health Care Management Review* 32: 203-
212.

Wilson, E., Chen, A.H., Wang, F., Fernandez, A. 2005. Effects of limited English proficiency and physician health care comprehension. *Journal of General Internal Medicine*. 20: 800-806.

World Health Organization. Prevention of hospital-acquired infections.

http://www.who.int/csr/resources/publications/whocdscsreph200212.pdf (accessed January 11, 2009).

Wrong Diagnosis. How common is misdiagnosis?î http://www.wrongdiagnosis.com/intro/common.htm (accessed January 10, 2009

Zhan, C. et., al. 2006. Medicare payment for selected adverse events: Building the business case for investing in patient safety. Health Affairs the Policy Journal of the Health Sphere 25(5): 1386-1393. http://content.healthaffairs.org/cgi/content/abstract/25/5/1386 (accessed April 26, 2009)